LAW AND ETHICS IN THE
PRACTICE OF PSYCHIATRY

AMERICAN COLLEGE OF PSYCHIATRISTS

Officers (at time of 1980 Annual Meeting)

SHERVERT H. FRAZIER, M.D., *President*

JOHN C. NEMIAH, M.D.
President-Elect

ROBERT L. WILLIAMS, M.D.
First Vice-President

HAROLD M. VISOTSKY, M.D.
Second Vice-President

HENRY H. WORK, M.D.
Secretary-General

CHARLES E. SMITH, M.D.
Treasurer

SIDNEY MALITZ, M.D.
Archivist-Historian

Program Committee for 1980 Annual Meeting

ALLAN BEIGEL, *Chairman*

KENNETH ALTSCHULER
JOHN DAVIS
JAMES EATON
PIETRO CASTELNUOVO-TEDESCO

RICHARD RADA
JACK BONNER
ROBERT O. PASNAU
GEORGE H. POLLOCK

Publications Committee

CHARLES HOFLING, *Chairman*

CARL EISDORFER
JOE YAMAMOTO
MICHAEL R. ZALES
JERRY M. LEWIS

RANSOM J. ARTHUR
HYMAN L. MUSLIN
HENRY H. WORK

Law and Ethics in the Practice of Psychiatry

Edited by

CHARLES K. HOFLING, M.D.

Professor of Psychiatry,
St. Louis University School of Medicine

BRUNNER/MAZEL, *Publishers* • New York

Library of Congress Cataloging in Publication Data

American College of Psychiatrists.
  Law and ethics in the practice of psychiatry.

  Papers presented at the 1980 annual meeting of the American College of Psychiatrists.
  Includes bibliographical references and index.
  1. Psychiatrists—Legal status, laws, etc.—United States.   2. Psychiatric ethics.   I. Hofling, Charles K.   II. Title.

KF2910.P75A45   174'.2   80-22091
ISBN 0-87630-250-9

Published by
BRUNNER/MAZEL, INC.
19 Union Square
New York, New York 10003

MANUFACTURED IN THE UNITED STATES OF AMERICA

A Tribute
CHARLES K. HOFLING, M.D.
1920-1980

Charles K. Hofling was killed in an automobile accident on May 17, 1980 in St. Louis, Missouri shortly after he finished writing the introduction to *Law and Ethics In the Practice of Psychiatry*. The last six months of his productive life were spent editing the material in this volume, a task he undertook with consummate skill and an abiding interest. In fact, his genius as an editor was in his shared enthusiasm with the writers for the work in progress.

As a member of the Publications Committee since 1969, Charles became involved in many of its publications. Particularly, he was co-editor with both Gene Usdin and Jerry Lewis of the two volumes preceding the current one. His interest in writing was catholic, ranging from articles on Shakespeare, Hardy, Hemingway, and Camus to textbooks on nursing. He was a fervent historian, and a renowned expert on American Indian culture.

His loss will be felt not only by the College, his friends and colleagues, his family, and his patients, but also by the world of letters. He was truly a "man for all seasons."

SHERVERT H. FRAZIER, M.D.
President, American College
of Psychiatrists

v

Contributors

ELISSA BENEDEK, M.D.

Director of Training and Education, Center for Forensic Psychiatry; Clinical Professor of Psychiatry, University of Michigan Medical Center, Ann Arbor

JEROME S. BEIGLER, M.D.

Clinical Professor of Psychiatry, University of Chicago, Pritzker School of Medicine, Chicago

PAUL CHODOFF, M.D.

Clinical Professor of Psychiatry, George Washington University, Washington, D. C.

GEORGE E. DIX, J.D.

Professor of Law, University of Texas at Austin

CAROL HABERMAN, LL.B.

Judge of the 45th District Court in San Antonio, Texas

JAY KATZ, M.D.

Professor of Law and Psychiatry, Yale Law School, New Haven, Connecticut

ROBERT MICHELS, M.D.

Barklie McKee Professor and Chairman, Department of Psychiatry, Cornell University Medical College; Psychiatrist-in-Chief, The New York Hospital, New York

RICHARD T. RADA, M.D.

Professor and Vice Chairman, Department of Psychiatry, School of Medicine, University of New Mexico, Albuquerque

JONAS RAPPEPORT, M.D.

Chief Medical Officer of the Supreme Bench of Baltimore, Baltimore, Maryland

NORMAN S. ROSENBERG, J.D.

Attorney and Co-Director, Developmental Disability Rights Center, Mental Health Law Project, Washington, D.C.

RALPH SLOVENKO, LL.B., Ph.D.

Professor of Law and Psychiatry, Wayne State University School of Law, Detroit, Michigan

JOHN SPECIA, LL.B.

Attorney for the Department of Human Resources, San Antonio, Texas

CAROL TUCKER, LL.B.

Attorney in Private Practice, San Antonio, Texas

WILLIAM J. WINSLADE, Ph.D., J.D.

Co-Director, The UCLA Program in Medicine, Law and Human Values, Los Angeles

Contents

ix

x   *Law and Ethics in the Practice of Psychiatry*

PART III
The Psychiatrist as an Expert Witness

PART IV
Ethical Issues

Introduction

One of the great stresses of a life in the practice of psychiatry is the continuing obligation to do the best one can in the face of ambiguity. Far overbalancing this consideration, however, is another one. Being basically concerned with the whole human organism—in other words, with *human nature*—the psychiatrist, to an extent unique among physicians, is involved in a continuous interplay with other major fields of human endeavor and concern. The biological sciences, the social sciences, the arts, the law, religion, and philosophy all have something to say to psychiatry, and all are capable of being, in some measure, integrated with the practice of psychiatry. The present volume, *Law and Ethics in the Practice of Psychiatry*, is one example of this breadth of common concerns.

This book is highly focused on practical issues, but is selective rather than comprehensive. For example, it is temporally selective. The past 20 years have seen a greatly increased interaction between psychiatry and the law, and this volume concentrates on some of the interfaces, such as issues of confidentiality and consent, that have become especially pressing and conspicuous. On ethical issues, the book also is selective. Certain issues—e.g., the conflict between psychiatry and religious value systems, a matter of clear ethical import—have largely subsided, and the present authors concentrate on such currently prominent ethical issues as the responsibilities of psychiatrists to society in various specific areas.

The chapters in this book fall rather naturally into an order of presentation. Part I is devoted to the development of necessary background material and the introduction of current issues and problems. In the first essay, Rosenberg traces the increased interaction between psychiatry and the law to two significant historical trends. The first of these is identified as a general awakening, or reawakening, of the public to serious problems in the delivery of mental health care, curiously concurrent with the growth of psychiatric authority. The second trend, now some 25 years old, is toward increased political and judicial activism. Against this background, the author closely considers two representative current issues: the right to treatment and the right to refuse treatment.

In an essay which is a marvel of organization and objectivity, Winslade traces the historical development of points of view, and ethical attitudes toward mental illness and mental health care since the last third of the 19th century. The author conveys a broad picture of an era as well as illustrating specific practices which exemplify it. Winslade divides his historical panorama into three periods: the Custodial (1870-1930), the Therapeutic (1930-1950), and the Systems Theory (1950-the present). He shows how pessimism and neglect gave way to a high but rather narrowly focused optimism, and the latter to an optimism tempered by realism but with a wider and more complex scope. The author, as befits his assignment, is not prescriptive, nor does he give the psychiatric reader a large amount of philosopical theory. He does show us the ethical presuppositions which have underlain—and currently underlie—psychiatric activities.

Part II of the book is devoted to a more thorough consideration of highly significant clinical issues. The three essays in this section are mutually supplementary. Beigler discusses problems of maintaining the necessary degree of privacy and confidentiality in the psychiatrist-patient relationship, problems which have, in our time, become critical as a result of four principal factors: the increasing involvement of third-party payers, the increasing threat of malpractice litigation, the trend (in some aspects, long-standing) of using psychiatrists as agents of social control, and the increasing demands of patients for access to their records.

The threats posed by these various pressures are well-documented and the author offers helpful suggestions for dealing with them constructively. Speaking unequivocally as a psychiatrist, Beigler discusses recent judicial and legislative developments which, in his view, "form a pattern of progressive erosions of the doctor-patient relationship so that clinical effectiveness is impaired and physicians are used as agents of police control" (p. 86).

In the following essay, Katz discusses the idea of disclosing relevant material to the psychiatric patient so that the latter's informed consent to—and a considerable degree of partnership in—the treatment enterprise can be obtained. The author clearly differentiates between an *idea* of this sort and a *doctrine* (legally sanctioned) and describes his efforts modestly as a quest for a doctrine. As suggested in his title, he is not certain that a thoroughly satisfactory doctrine is achievable. If it proves to be so, the considerations shared in this essay may well be essential to that end. This clearly written essay is both subtle and profound, setting forth the perspectives of law, medicine, and psychiatry, and then concentrating on issues pertaining to the last-mentioned discipline. The discussion of transference and countertransference is particularly helpful.

All the mental health professions, and particularly psychiatry, have been disturbingly stimulated, even shaken, by the celebrated *Tarasoff* decision and its possible implications. In the concluding essay of this section, Dix thoroughly discusses the *Tarasoff* decicision. The discussion is probing, thorough and non-dogmatic. The *Tarasoff* decision is spelled out, its ramifications are explored, its impact on the disclosures of a therapist requisite for the obtaining of informed consent is considered, and the basic question of policy—should a *Tarasoff*-type liability persist?—is discussed. Finally, there is a consideration of possible alternative doctrines. Throughout the essay, there is the sense of a sustained intellectual encounter between author and reader.

Part III brings together the psychiatrist and the law. Rada's paper considers the psychiatrist as an expert witness. The author delineates this role which may vary, at times involving testimony limited to medical facts and at other times involving an expert opinion drawn from such facts. The differences in the psychiatrist's serving as an expert for the plaintiff, for the defendant, or for the court are clarified. The limitations of the psychiatrist's role are explained by way of contrasting it with those of the judge, the jury, and the attorneys. Preparations for testifying are described: preparation as to attitude, knowledge, and courtroom skills. Important pitfalls for the psychiatrist to avoid are described—not merely the obvious pitfalls resulting from inadequate preparation, but the subtler ones deriving from unconscious biases (i.e., "countertransference"). Rada concludes that the special requirements of giving expert testimony indicate that this role is not for every psychiatrist, but that, with attention to the considerations presented, it can be constructively handled by most.

Slovenko presents, in an even-handed and detailed way, the issues and presumptions involved in child custody cases. He points out some of the factors which are currently making for more frequent and more complex disputes than have hitherto been the case, including "no-fault divorce" and the greater emancipation of women. The best interests of the child have for some time been a substantial issue in these cases, having supplanted the old "parental-right" doctrine, but the author stresses the problems of evaluation and decision which have grown with the newer emphasis on psychological welfare. Pertinent legislation has been developed, and Slovenko cites highly illustrative material from various states. The author concludes that the relevant issues, in the assessment of which psychiatrists play a significant part, are far from being generally and satisfactorily settled.

The balance of Part III brings to life the material in the Rada and Slovenko essays. The technical device used is a mock-trial demonstration, involving psychiatric testimony on a question of child custody, with introductory remarks by Rada and with Judge Haberman of San Antonio, Texas, presiding. The transcription speaks for itself, and it should be stressed that the material is presented essentially verbatim, as it was heard at the American College of Psychiatrists meeting.

Part IV is devoted to a presentation of certain specific ethical issues facing psychiatrists individually and collectively: namely, their responsibilities to today's society. As is true of the other contributors to this volume, the authors do not become deeply theoretical. They do, however, examine the issues closely and their premises are, so far as this editor knows, shared by most other thoughtful American psychiatrists.

In the first of these papers, Chodoff considers the responsibilities of the individual psychiatrist to society. He lists the basic components of this responsibility as the general ones of a concerned citizen, as accountability to the public, and as an unselfish willingness to promote the provision of services to all those in need of them. Issues such as the conflict between loyalty to a less-than-competent colleague and concern for the welfare of patients, the profession, and the public, and the conflict between accountability to patients and that to third-party payers, are assessed with delicacy and candor.

In the companion paper, Michels shifts the focus from the responsibilities of the individual psychiatrist to those of the profession as a whole. After a helpful introductory section on professions and professionalism in general, the author turns to the ethical questions facing psychiatry. His standards are high, and he endorses the time-tested (but too often ignored) truth that "science cannot tell us which goal to pursue first and which to defer or even relinquish" (p. 243). The acquisition of knowledge, the careful selection and conscientious, nonexploitive education of trainees, and the monitoring of the quality of professional work are examples of the demands which the profession of psychiatry faces.

This American College of Psychiatrists' volume endeavors to set forth a representative and balanced view of legal and ethical issues confronting psychiatry today, not minimizing difficulties or differences, but indicating ways in which psychiatry can utilize knowledge from law and ethics.

CHARLES K. HOFLING, M.D.

LAW AND ETHICS IN THE PRACTICE OF PSYCHIATRY

Part I

HISTORICAL PERSPECTIVES

1

Law and the Mental Health System: The Challenge of Change

Norman S. Rosenberg, J.D.

INTRODUCTION

The extent of interaction between psychiatry and law is greater today than anyone could have imagined a decade ago. The role of psychiatrists in the legal system was then largely confined to providing testimony in insanity defense and civil commitment proceedings. Now, psychiatrists routinely find themselves involved in a wide range of legal issues, including procedural safeguards in the civil commitment process, standards of adequate patient care, privacy and confidentiality, informed consent, and institutional accountability.

Lawyers, too, have noted a change, with the emergence of a discrete mental health bar in the last 10 years. Public interest organizations, such as the Mental Health Law Project, have been created with the express purpose of addressing the complex is-

The views expressed in this article are those of the author and do not necessarily reflect the views or policies of the Mental Health Law Project. The author's work is partially supported by a grant from the Foundation for Child Development.

sues at the intersection of law and the behavioral sciences. Attorneys specializing in representation of mentally ill and developmentally disabled persons have joined legal aid programs and
formed patient advocacy offices; state mental health departments
have employed more lawyers; and growing numbers of private
practitioners list mental health law among their areas of spe-
cialization.

Other examples of cross-disciplinary dialogue and specializa-
tion abound. The American Bar Association has created a special
Commission on the Mentally Disabled. The American Psychiatric
Association (APA) has a Commission on Judicial Action. Inter-
disciplinary organizations such as the American Academy of Psychiatry and Law have been formed, and distinguished professional and scholarly associations, such as the American College
of Psychiatrists, have devoted annual meetings, conferences, and
symposia to the study of mental health law issues, the patients'
rights movement, and related topics of mutual interest and
concern.

HISTORICAL OVERVIEW

Considered in the context of two historical trends, the increased interaction between psychiatry and the law was perhaps
inevitable. The first of these trends is a recent reawakening interest in the problems that have plagued the mental health
delivery system since the mid-19th century and concern with the
growth of psychiatric authority during this period. The second
trend is the political and judicial activism that surfaced in the
United States in the late 1950s.

Psychiatry in the first half of the 19th century was marked by
great enthusiasm and optimism. A "cult of curability" captivated
the profession during those years (1). Reportedly high rates of
cure of mental illness sparked a movement by liberal progressives
to draw distinctions between mentally ill persons and criminals.
The former were deemed worthy of and amenable to treatment,
the latter not (2). This assumption led to the development of a
civil commitment system which purported to treat the mentally

ill. It also translated into a dramatic expansion in the authority of medical professionals as courts abdicated their decision-making role to psychiatrists (3). This authority was and continues to be ill-defined and without effective limitation, and, for the most part, psychiatrists do not recognize the potential for its abuse (4).

By the mid-20th century, an extraordinary number of people were involuntarily confined in mental institutions. However, treatment methodologies were limited, financial resources inadequate, and discriminatory commitment procedures led to the hospitalization of politically underrepresented groups—immigrants, the poor, racial minorities, the aged, and the mentally retarded. As a result, state hospitals acquired and maintained a reputation as warehouses—places where people were incarcerated for life (5).

The state hospital system has never had a constituency in the middle class and has never gained substantial public support (6). However, periodic disclosures by the media of the intolerable conditions that existed in these institutions, particularly after World War II, generated public calls for change. At the same time, contemporary mental health theory and research began to support the view that large institutions were inherently bad (7) and that they created more problems of chronicity than they cured (8). Critics began to suggest that the entire mental health enterprise was ideologically corrupt (9) and that the mentally ill were simply the scapegoats of society (10).

In the late 1950s through the 1960s, while public cries for reform of the mental health system were going unanswered, the United States was embroiled in a social revolution aimed at securing basic civil and human rights for racial minorities, the criminally accused, and other disadvantaged groups. The era was marked by judicial activism unparalleled in recent history and by dramatic expansion of services and programs for the poor, including legal services—described by some observers as the most successful component of Lyndon Johnson's "War on Poverty" (11). Frustrated by the persistent failure of traditional social pressures to bring about reforms in the mental health system and inspired by the impressive victories earned by poverty lawyers, professional organizations and patients formed a loose coalition with lawyers to establish and enforce the rights of mentally disabled persons, primarily through the use of litigation. This coalition has been the catalyst for what has been described as a "revolutionary" patients' rights movement (12). During the 1970s, this group was responsible for securing important rights for mental patients, including: the right to treatment (13), protection from harm (14), the right to treatment in the "least restrictive setting" (15), equal educational opportunity (16), protection from forced administration of hazardous or intrusive therapeutic procedures (17), the right to procedural and substantive safeguards in the commitment process (18), and the right to liberty (19).

From the perspective of patients' rights lawyers, the victories achieved have been dramatic and impressive, but they have not been won without cost. One of these costs has been the ideological confrontation that has emerged between the mental health and legal systems. I will explore this confrontation in the context of two of the key issues addressed by the patients' rights movement to date: the right to treatment and the right to refuse treatment.

THE RIGHT TO TREATMENT

The first case addressing the right to treatment which evoked national attention was *Rouse v. Cameron* (20). Rouse had been committed to Saint Elizabeth's Hospital in Washington, D.C. in 1962, after having been found not guilty, by reason of insanity, of possessing a dangerous weapon—a misdemeanor carrying a one-year maximum sentence. After three years of hospitalization, Rouse petitioned for release on the grounds that he had not received psychiatric treatment during this period. The trial court dismissed his claim, but the court of appeals reversed and remanded the case. Appellate Judge David Bazelon's opinion declared: "The purpose of involuntary hospitalization is treatment, not punishment. . . . Absent treatment, the hospital is transform[ed] . . . into a penitentiary where one could be held indefinitely for no convicted offense" (21).

Although the court's decision was based upon interpretation of a District of Columbia statute, it strongly implied that a constitutional right to treatment exists under the due process, equal protection, and cruel and unusual punishment clauses. The court stated:

> Absence of treatment might draw into question the constitutionality of this mandatory commitment section. . . . It has also been suggested that failure to supply treatment may violate the equal protection clause. Indefinite confinement without treatment of one who has been found not criminally responsible may be so inhumane as to be cruel and unusual punishment (22).

While *Rouse* was greeted euphorically by reform-minded advocates, who viewed the decision as a step toward improving the deplorable conditions that existed in state hospitals, the psychiatric profession was noticeably less enthusiastic. It viewed the decision as an unwarranted intrusion into its professional domain. This concern was highlighted in the American Psychiatric Association's official response to the decision. The Council of APA declared:

> The definition of treatment and the appraisal of its adequacy are matters for medical determination. . . . The conceptual contrasting of "treatment" on the one hand with "punishment" on the other sometimes obfuscates more than it clarifies the problem. Some courts, attorneys, statutes, and judicial formulations reiterate, almost ritualistically, that hospitalization without treatment equates with punishment. This is not precisely the case (23).

Although *Rouse* was an important legal victory, as a practical matter it represented a very minor encroachment on the autonomy of the psychiatric profession. Five years later, however, the patients' rights movement took a giant leap forward with the court's decision in *Wyatt v. Stickney* (24). In *Wyatt* the nascent right-to-treatment principle emerged as a fundamental legal doctrine.

Wyatt began as a class action brought by patients and staff of

Alabama's Bryce Hospital. The case sought an injunction to prevent the state from carrying through its plan to dismiss a substantial number of employees because of budgetary reductions (25). However, after personally touring the hospital and after taking testimony from expert witnesses as to the environmental and personnel resources that are minimally necessary for treatment to take place, Judge Frank M. Johnson, Jr. declared the entire hospital setting to be an unconstitutional deprivation of the patients' right to treatment (26). He articulated the constitutional principle underlying the court's decision as follows:

> There can be no legal (or moral) justification for the state of Alabama's failing to afford treatment . . . to the several thousand patients who have been civilly committed . . . for treatment purposes. To deprive any citizen of his or her liberty upon the altruistic theory that the confinement is for humane and therapeutic reasons and then fail to provide adequate treatment violates the very fundamentals of due process (27).

The court then conducted a three-day hearing before entering its final order. Several of the major professional associations, including the American Psychological Association, the American Orthopsychiatric Association, and the American Association on Mental Deficiency, participated in those hearings as *amici curiae*. The American Psychiatric Association did not.

In April 1972, the court issued its order, the most significant ruling in the evolution of the right-to-treatment movement. It promulgated a detailed set of standards for adequate treatment, governing virtually every aspect of institutional care from environmental conditions to the patient's basic right to privacy, from staffing ratios to limitations on the administration of medication (28). Anticipating fiscal arguments against fulfilling the terms of the decree, the court stated that "the unavailability of neither funds, nor staff nor facilities, will justify a default by defendants in the provision of suitable treatment" (29).

The *Wyatt* decision exposed dramatically the hypocrisy of the civil commitment process and the substandard conditions which existed in Alabama's not atypical hospitals. Under the guise of benevolence, deviant members of society were being arbitrarily removed from their homes and communities and placed on the back wards of large, remote institutions, where they languished for life without adequate care or treatment.

While the objectives of the *Wyatt* litigation have been widely applauded, and while APA eventually supported the plaintiffs' position when the state appealed the decision, the court's decree has met with repeated criticism from various segments of the psychiatric profession. One of the major criticisms is that the only feasible way to measure the adequacy of treatment is against the needs of a particular patient (30). The court's standards are, therefore, not enforceable, because it is neither practical nor possible for courts to monitor the delivery of adequate services to each patient. Another criticism states that treatment is a term encompassing so many approaches that defining its adequacy can only be a post hoc judgment made without regard for the actual choices faced by the medical staff (31).

These objections have been addressed by Alan Stone in his NIMH monograph, *Mental Health and Law: A System in Transition* (32). Stone points out that, although it is true that each patient in a hospital has a right to adequate treatment, even those courts most supportive of the right-to-treatment principle acknowledge that the right does not adhere to the single, hypothetically best treatment, but merely to "adequate treatment" (33), a bona fide effort to help the patient—to afford him a realistic opportunity to improve or be cured. Thus, in determining whether a hospital has made sufficient efforts to treat and cure its patients, the role of the court appears similar to the role it assumes in reviewing agency actions and other matters of equal complexity (34). In this context, the court might review the extent of a hospital's effort by hearing expert testimony regarding whether the patient has received that degree of a mode of therapy which some reputable segment of the profession deems appropriate. Furthermore, although it is true that opinions are quite diverse as to appropriate treatment modalities, when no treatment of any kind is offered, there is little argument. For example, in *Wyatt*, Judge Johnson made it clear that the court's role was not to choose between various arguably effective therapeutic modalities, but rather to eliminate the conditions which made effective treatment impossible (35).

Psychiatrists have at least one further concern with the *Wyatt* case and other litigation in the mental disabilities area. While it is not often expressed publicly, I believe that the psychiatric profession is concerned with the extent to which courts rather than mental health professionals have the power and responsibility for defining and measuring the adequacy of services provided to mentally disabled persons (36). Because of fears of loss of power and professional autonomy and because of concerns regarding their liability for decisions over which they have little or no control, psychiatrists and other mental health professionals are alarmed by the growing tendency of lawyers and judges to substitute their judgment for that of the professionals (37). Indeed, the legal and sociological literature is strewn with complaints of "overdoses of due process" (38) and stories of patients "dying with their rights on" (39). In this context, it is easy to see how a challenge to professional discretion such as this one increases psychiatrists' resentment of the legal process. Such resentment is likely to be intensified if these same psychiatrists are held personally liable for their actions. In fact, this was precisely the outcome of the Supreme Court's historic decision in *O'Connor v. Donaldson* (40).

Kenneth Donaldson had been civilly committed and confined at the Florida State Hospital at Chattahoochee for 14 years, when he sued state hospital psychiatrists for money damages pursuant to the Civil Rights Act (41), alleging that members of the hospital staff had intentionally and maliciously deprived him of his constitutional right to liberty. After a four-day trial, a Florida jury awarded Donaldson $38,500 in compensatory and punitive damages (42) against two psychiatrists who had served as director of the ward in which Donaldson resided and clinical director of the hospital. The psychiatrists appealed, contending that the Constitution does not guarantee a right to treatment to involuntarily committed mental patients. After the appeal was denied by the Fifth Circuit Court of Appeals, the defendants petitioned the United States Supreme Court.

On June 26, 1975, the Supreme Court unanimously declared that Donaldson's right to liberty had been violated. Interestingly, the Supreme Court made no finding in the case—nor has it in any other—that there is or is not a constitutional right to treatment. The Court stated:

> There is no reason now to decide whether mentally ill persons dangerous to themselves or to others have a right to treatment upon compulsory confinement by the State, or whether the State may compulsorily confine a nondangerous, mentally ill individual for the purpose of treatment (43).

As the case was presented, neither issue had to be resolved. The Court viewed the case as one which raised the simple but nonetheless important question concerning an individual's constitutional right to liberty. On this issue, the Court stated:

> A finding of "mental illness" alone cannot justify a State's locking a person up against his will and keeping him indefinitely in simple custodial confinement. . . . There is still no constitutional basis for confining such persons involuntarily if they are dangerous to no one and can live safely in freedom (44).

As psychiatrists faced the stark reality that they could be held personally liable for monetary damages when patient care and treatment fell below judicially determined standards, predictions swiftly followed of the demise of the state mental hospital system (45). While those ominous forecasts proved unfounded, the case surely exacerbated tensions which intensified further as the patients' rights movement approached a new, controversial vista—the effort to establish the right to refuse treatment.

THE RIGHT TO REFUSE TREATMENT

The institutionalized patient's right to refuse treatment is an issue of enormous complexity, involving legal, medical, psychological, and ethical considerations. It has been the focus of considerable scholarly attention (46). Psychiatrists are especially sensitive about this issue because it questions the greatly expanded authority which has accrued to the profession in recent years. The stakes in this controversy are undeniably high. At issue are the nature and extent of limitations upon the psychiatrist's power to impose treatment procedures upon unwilling or incompetent persons.

The Legal Analytic Framework

The legal analytic framework in support of the right to refuse treatment stems from a composite of bases, including the common law protection against unwanted intentional contact with one's body (47), constitutional rights to freedom from harm, freedom of speech and thought, and personal privacy (48), as well as state statutes and administrative regulations promulgated to regulate treatment procedures within a state system or within a particular institution (49). This framework has been fully described in the literature (50) and will not be repeated here. For the purposes of this discussion suffice it to say that the fundamental principle underlying these bases is that no patient may be forced to accept treatment without his or her informed consent. For consent to be valid, it must be competent, knowledgeable, and voluntary (51). As explained by the court in a celebrated psychosurgery case, *Kaimowitz v. Michigan Department of Mental Health* (52), this means:

> The involuntarily detained mental patient must have legal capacity to give consent (that is, the ability to rationally understand the nature of the procedure, its risks and other relevant information). He must be so situated as to be able to exercise free power of choice without any element of force, fraud, deceit, duress, overreaching, or other ulterior form of restraint or coercion. He must have sufficient knowledge and comprehension of the subject matter to enable him to make an understanding decision.

The application of the principle of informed consent to a person who is civilly committed because, for example, he is dangerous to himself or others by reason of mental illness, has created challenging problems for treatment professionals and has generated considerable conflict between lawyers and psychiatrists. To a large extent, the conflict derives from a disparity between the legal effect of a civil commitment determination and the practical assumptions underlying it.

Under most commitment laws in this country, an individual's legal competency is not at issue. Therefore, a decision to civilly commit someone does not mean, as a matter of law, that that person has been determined incompetent. Moreover, it is now generally recognized that people who are committable may have impaired functioning in some areas but be perfectly functional and competent in others. For example, as the court noted in *Winters v. Miller* (53):

> The law is quite clear in New York that a finding of "mental illness" even by a judge or jury, and commitment to a hospital, does not raise even a presumption that the patient is "incompetent" or unable adequately to manage his own affairs. Absent a specific finding of incompetence, the mental patient retains the right to sue or defend in his own name, to sell or dispose of his property, to marry, draft a will, and in general to manage his own affairs (54).

As a practical matter, however, once institutionalized, patients are treated as though they are not competent. Indeed, whether a person voluntarily signs himself into a hospital or is committed pursuant to a court order, it is widely assumed by hospital administrators and staff that they have the authority to treat the patient in whatever manner they deem appropriate (55).

From the civil liberties perspective, such attitudes are obviously untenable. By the same token, most psychiatrists strongly believe that recognizing every patient's right to refuse treatment, no matter how disturbed or disoriented the patient may be, is an ill-conceived expansion of the concept of personal autonomy.

To date there have been comparatively few cases concerning the right to refuse treatment. However, those which have been decided have attempted to mediate between the two extreme positions. A notable recent example is *Rogers v. Okin* (56), decided in October, 1979, by a federal district court in Massachusetts. This class action lawsuit alleged that the defendants, doctors at the Boston State Hospital, maintained policies of forced medication and involuntary seclusion of patients, in violation of their constitutional rights.

Attorneys representing patients at Boston State theorized that, although the patients had a right to receive treatment when confined at a state mental institution, they also had a constitutional right to refuse such treatment. They acknowledged that such a right to refuse was not absolute—that it must be weighed against the hospital's right to impose treatment in order to protect the safety of both patients and staff. At the same time, the plaintiffs insisted that, except in emergency circumstances, they were competent to decide whether or not to accept treatment, and that their decision must be respected by hospital physicians. Following a 72-day trial which included testimony by more than 50 witnesses, most of whom were psychiatrists, psychologists, and other professionals, the court issued its long-awaited ruling.

Holding that both voluntarily and involuntarily confined patients have a right to refuse medication, absent an emergency situation, Judge Joseph L. Tauro declared:

> It is an unreasonable invasion of privacy, and an affront to basic concepts of human dignity, to permit forced injection of mind-altering drugs into the buttocks of a competent patient unwilling to give informed consent. . . .
>
> Given the alternatives available in non-emergencies, subjecting a patient to the humiliation of being disrobed and then injected with drugs powerful enough to immobilize both body and mind is totally unreasonable by any standard. Forced injections in non-emergencies are classic intrusions which are not justified in the circumstances (57).

Both parties in the suit had agreed that a constitutional right to refuse treatment could be overridden in emergency circumstances. Therefore, the definition of what constituted an emergency became a key disputed issue in the litigation. Significantly, the court's decision rejected the defendants' proposed standard for determining when an emergency existed. In the doctors' view, a "psychiatric emergency" justifying forced medication existed under any of the following circumstances: 1) suicidal behavior, whether seriously meant or a gesture; 2) assaultiveness; 3) property destruction; 4) extreme anxiety and panic; 5) bizarre behavior; 6) acute or chronic emotional disturbance having the potential to seriously interfere with the patient's ability to function on a daily basis; and 7) the necessity for immediate medical response in order to prevent or decrease the likelihood of further severe suffering or the rapid worsening of the patient's clinical state.

The court called this definition "too broad, subjective and unwieldy" (58), and declared that:

> The fact that a set of circumstances may fall within the broad parameters of a psychiatric emergency does not necessarily justify any and all responsive steps taken thereafter by a doctor. . . .

> This court holds, therefore, that a committed mental patient may be forcibly medicated in an emergency situation in which a failure to do so would result in a *substantial likelihood of physical harm* to that patient, other patients, or to staff members of the institution (59). (Emphasis added.)

In *Rogers,* the court attempted to strike a balance between two important interests, the private right of patients—both voluntary and involuntarily committed but legally competent—to refuse medication, and the state's interest in treating patients who present an imminent danger to themselves or others, or who are incompetent to provide consent to treatment. For the most part, the court's solution is a reasonable accommodation of these interests. However, the *Rogers* framework, like other models which have been proposed in recent years (60), imposes clear restraints on psychiatrists' far-reaching discretion in treatment decisions. Not surprisingly, then, the psychiatric establishment is troubled both by the decision itself and the trend of which it is a part.

Some courts have also expressed concern that judicial scrutiny of psychiatrists' decisions will interfere with necessary treatment and will render such treatment more expensive and time-consuming. For example, in *Parham v. J.L.* (61), in rejecting the requirement of an evidentiary hearing prior to the admission of a child to a mental hospital, the Supreme Court stated:

> The State also has a genuine interest in allocating priority to the diagnosis and treatment of patients. . . . One factor that must be considered is the utilization of the time of psychiatrists, psychologists and other behavioral specialists in preparing for and participating in hearings rather than performing the task for which their special training has fitted them. Behavioral experts in courtrooms and hearings are of little help to patients (61).

While the *Parham* decision is distinguishable from Rogers in many respects—*e.g., Parham* involved the complex question of the scope of process due to a child whose commitment is proposed initially by the parent—the Court's decision, nevertheless, evidences a clear interest in shielding psychiatric decisions from judicial oversight.

The balance between the legal right to refuse treatment and sound medical judgment is a delicate one which does not lend itself to simplistic solutions. However, in light of the misunderstanding and distrust that have polarized the psychiatric and legal professions as a result of this issue, it may be useful to convey my sense of the objectives and direction of the patients' rights movement. In attempting to establish minimum requirements for the use of extraordinary or potentially hazardous modes of treatment, including somatic therapies such as psychotropic medications, lawyers and judges are bent neither on stripping psychiatrists of their authority nor on tying their hands in the treatment room. Diagnostic decisions are a medical judgment and are acknowledged as being outside the province or expertise of the legal system. However, questions of compulsion and intrusion on the autonomy of both voluntary and involuntarily committed patients are fundamentally legal questions and are legitimately the concern of lawyers, courts, and legislatures (62). For this reason, lawyers will continue to pursue judicial scrutiny of involuntarily imposed treatment and the establishment of appropriate procedural and substantive safeguards accompanying such procedures when administered to both competent and incompetent persons. Unfortunately, in the present climate, each such challenge will probably exacerbate tensions in an area that, in the words of Harold Lasswell, "sorely needs a reduction in provocation" (63).

CONCLUSION

The movements to establish the right to treatment and the right to refuse treatment have resulted in considerable tension between lawyers seeking to establish controls on psychiatric decision-making and mental health professionals resisting the imposition of legal regulation. There are other confrontations between these disciplines on a daily basis—for example, challenges to psychiatric expertise regarding patients' needs for continued institutionalization and in predicting dangerousness in the civil commitment context, and efforts to regulate misuse and dissemination of patient treatment records and to ensure patient access to such records.

The sketch that I have drawn could lead to the pessimistic conclusion that the two professions are locked in a struggle which threatens their capacity for collaboration and compromise and may even jeopardize effective patient care. But I do not believe this is so. Reconstructing the history of the patients' rights movement, one is reminded that it evolved from an alliance, not only of patients, lawyers, and consumer groups, but of psychiatrists, psychologists, social workers, and the leading mental health professional associations. Even today, as success in eradicating the intolerable conditions which existed in many institutions a decade ago has afforded us the luxury of shifting our focus to more subtle and complex issues—issues, such as the right to refuse treatment, that may involve challenges to the judgments of psychiatrists—many distinguished psychiatrists continue to be among the most ardent and constructive supporters of the patients' rights movement.

Obviously, our perspectives and opinions regarding such issues will not always be congruent. The tension between legal controls and mental health treatment goals stems from divergent ethical, political and economic considerations which will surely exist for years to come. As a result, the legal and psychiatric professions will periodically find themselves in antagonistic positions—on opposite sides of the issues and of the courtroom. Despite these disputes, lawyers and psychiatrists should not lose sight of the host of issues in which their interests merge on behalf of mentally disabled persons. The challenge facing us today is to develop and maintain a climate in which collaboration around these issues may continue.

REFERENCES

1. Deutsch, A.: *The Mentally Ill in America.* New York: Columbia University Press, 1949, 132-157.
2. Halleck, S.: American Psychiatry and the Criminal: A Historical Review. *American Journal of Psychiatry,* 121 (1965), Supplement, i-xxi, at v.
3. Stone, A.: *Mental Health and Law: A System in Transition.* Washington, D.C.: USDHEW, 1975, p. 1.
4. Robitscher, J.: The Limits of Psychiatric Authority. *International Journal of Law and Psychiatry,* 1:183-204, 1973.
5. *See, e.g.,* Grob, G. N.: *The State and the Mentally Ill.* Chapel Hill, N.C.: University of North Carolina Press, 1966; Rothman, D. J.: *The Discovery of the Asylum.* Boston: Little, Brown & Co., 1971.
6. Levine, M.: *From State Hospital to Psychiatric Center.* The Harlem Valley Psychiatric Center, December 31, 1978 (unpublished).
7. *See, e.g.,* Goffman, E.: *Asylums.* Garden City, N.Y.: Doubleday, 1971; Joint Commission on Mental Health and Illness: *Action for Mental Health.* New York: John Wiley & Sons, 1961.
8. *See, e.g.,* Scheff, T. J.: *Being Mentally Ill.* Chicago: Aldine, 1966.
9. Szasz, T.: *Law, Liberty and Psychiatry.* New York: Macmillan & Co., 1963.
10. Szasz, T.: *The Myth of Mental Illness.* New York: Dell Publishing Co., 1961.
11. Wald, P. and Friedman, P.: The Politics of Mental Health Advocacy in the United States. *International Journal of Law and Psychiatry,* 1: 137-152, 1978.
12. *Ibid.*
13. *Rouse v. Cameron,* 373 F.2d 451 (D.C. Cir. 1966); *Wyatt v. Stickney,* 325 F. Supp. 781, 784 (M.D. Ala. 1971), 334 F. Supp. 1341 (M.D. Ala. 1971), 344 F. Supp. 373 and 387 (M.D. Ala 1972), *aff'd sub nom. Wyatt v. Aderholt,* 503 F.2d 1305 (5th Cir. 1974); *Welsch v. Likins,* 373 F. Supp.

487, 493 (D. Minn. 1974); *Davis v. Watkins*, 384 F. Supp. 1196, 1203-12 (N.D. Ohio 1974); *Gary W. v. Cherry sub nom. Gary W. v. Louisiana*, 437 F. Supp. 1209 (E.D. La. 1976).

14. *E.g.*, *New York State Association for Retarded Children, Inc. v. Rockefeller*, 357 F. Supp. 752, 764 (E.D.N.Y. 1973), consent judgment approved *sub nom. New York State Association for Retarded Children, Inc. v. Carey*, 393 F. Supp. 715 (E.D.N.Y. 1975).
15. *E.g.*, *Dixon v. Weinberger*, 405 F. Supp. 974 (D.D.C. 1975).
16. *E.g.*, *Pennsylvania Association for Retarded Children v. Pennsylvania*, 334 F. Supp. 1257 (E.D. Pa. 1971), 343 F. Supp. 279 (E.D. Pa. 1972); *Mills v. Board of Education*, 348 F. Supp. 866 (D.D.C. 1972).
17. *E.g.*, *Kaimowitz v. Michigan Department of Mental Health*, Civil No. 73-19434-AW, 42 U.S.L.W. 2063 (Mich. Cir. Ct. 1973); *Scott v. Plante*, 532 F.2d 939, 946 (3d Cir. 1976); *Rennie v. Klein*, 462 F. Supp. 1131 (D.N.J. 1978); *Rogers v. Okin*, No. 75-1610-T (D. Mass. 1979).
18. *E.g.*, *Lessard v. Schmidt*, 349 F. Supp. 1078 (E.D. Wis. 1972); *Lynch v. Baxley*, 386 F. Supp. 378 (M.D. Ala. 1974); *Bell v. Wayne County General Hospital*, 384 F. Supp. 1085 (E.D. Mich. 1975).
19. *O'Connor v. Donaldson*, 422 U.S. 563 (1975).
20. *Rouse, supra* note 13.
21. *Ibid.*, at 452-53.
22. *Ibid.*, at 453.
23. Council of the American Psychiatric Association, Position Paper on the Question of Adequacy of Treatment. *American Journal of Psychiatry*, 123:1458, 1967.
24. *Wyatt, supra* note 13, 325 F. Supp. 781 (M.D. Ala. 1971).
25. *Fremouw*, W. J.: A New Right to Treatment. In Golann, S. and Fremouw, W. J. (Eds.), *The Right to Treatment for Mental Patients*. New York: Irvington Publishers, Inc., 1976.
26. *Wyatt, supra* note 13, 325 F. Supp. 781 (M.D. Ala. 1971).
27. *Ibid.* at 785.
28. *Wyatt, supra* note 13, 344 F. Supp. 373 and 387 (M.D. Ala. 1972).
29. *Ibid.*, at 377.
30. *See, e.g., Burnham v. Department of Mental Health*, 349 F. Supp. 1335, 1343 (N.D. Ga. 1972).
31. Szasz, T.: The Right to Health. 49 Geo. L.J. 734 (1967).
32. *Supra* note 3.
33. *Millard v. Cameron*, 373 F.2d 468, 472 (D.C. Cir. 1968).
34. Bazelon, D. L.: Implementing the Right to Treatment, 36 *U. of Chicago L. Rev.* 742-54 (1969).
35. *Wyatt, supra* note 13, 344 F. Supp. 373, 375-76 (M.D. Ala. 1972).
36. *See, e.g.*, Rosenberg, N. and Friedman, P.: Developmental Disability Law: A Look Into the Future, 31 *Stanford L. Rev.* 817 (1979).
37. Roos, P.: The Law and Mentally Retarded People: An Uncertain Future, 31 *Stanford L Rev.* 619 (1979).
38. Rachlin: One Right Too Many. *3 Bull. Am. Acad. Psychiatry & L.*, 95 (1975).
39. Treffert, D.: Dying With Their Rights On. *Prism*, Feb. 1974, at 47.
40. *Supra* note 19.

41. 42 U.S.C. § 1983.
42. The jury award was ultimately vacated and remanded by the Supreme Court. Donaldson eventually received a damages settlement of $20,000.
43. *Supra* note 19, at 573.
44. *Ibid.*, at 575.
45. *See, e.g.,* Stone, A.: The Right to Treatment and the Psychiatric Establishment. *Psychiatric Annals* 4:9, 1974.
46. *See, e.g., Friedman,* P.: Legal Regulation of Applied Behavior Analysis in Mental Institutions, 17 *Arizona L. Rev.* 39 (1975); Comment, Informed Consent and the Mental Patient's Right to Refuse Psychosurgery and Shock Treatment, 75 *Mich. L. Rev.* 363 (1976); Bomstein, M.: The Forcible Administration of Drugs to Prisoners and Mental Patients, 9 *Clearinghouse Rev.* 379 (1975); Stone, A.: The Right of the Psychiatric Patient to Refuse Treatment, 4 *J. Psych. & Law* 515 (1976); Perlin, M.: The Right to Refuse Treatment in New Jersey, 6 *Psych. Annals* 300 (1976); Brooks, A.: The Right to Refuse Treatment, *Administration in Mental Health,* Vol. 4, 90 (1977); Gaughan and LaRue: The Right of a Mental Patient to Refuse Antipsychotic Drugs in an Institution, 4 *Law and Psychology Rev.* 43 (1978); Plotkin, R.: Limiting the Therapeutic Orgy: Mental Patients' Right to Refuse Treatment, 72 *Northwestern U. L. Rev.* 461 (1977).
47. *See, generally,* Prosser, W., Law of Torts, § 10, 18, 32 (4th ed. 1971).
48. *See, e.g., Rozecki v. Gaughan,* 459 F.2d 6 (1st Cir. 1972); *Mackey v. Procunier,* 477 F.2d 877 (9th Cir. 1973); *Kaimowitz v. Michigan Dept. of Mental Health, supra* note 17.
49. *See, e.g.,* N.Y. Mental Hygiene Law §15.03 (b) (4) (McKinney Supp. 1974-75); N.J. Statutes Annotated 30:4-24.1 and 24.2 (1975).
50. *Supra* note 46.
51. *See, e.g.,* Waltz and Scheuneman, Informed Consent to Therapy. 64 *Northwestern U.L. Rev.* 628 (1970); Comment, Informed Consent in Medical Malpractice. 55 *Cal. L. Ref.* 1396 (1967).
52. *Supra* note 17, at 2063-64.
53. *See Winters v. Miller,* 446 F.2d 65 (2d Cir.), *cert. denied,* 404 U.S. 985 (1971); *Henry v. Cicerone,* 315 F. Supp. 889 (W.D. Mo. 1970).
54. *Winters v. Miller, supra* note 73, at 68.
55. Brooks, A.: *Law, Psychiatry and the Mental Health System* 877 (1974).
56. 478 F. Supp. 1342 (1979).
57. *Ibid.*, at 1369.
58. *Ibid.*, at 1365.
59. *Ibid.*
60. *See, e.g.,* Stone, A., *supra* note 3, at 104-106; Legal Issues in State Mental Health Care: Proposals for Change, in 2 *Mental Disability Law Reporter* (1977); President's Commission on Mental Health, Report of the Task Panel on Legal and Ethical Issues, in 20 *Arizona L. Rev.* 49, 109-110 (1978).
61. *Parham v. J.L.,* 99 S. Ct. 2493, 47 U.S.L.W. 4740 (June 20, 1979).
62. *See, e.g., Wyatt v. Hardin,* Unpublished Order, Civil No. 3195-N (M.D. Ala., Feb. 28, 1975).
63. Lasswell, H.: *Power and Personality.* New York: Viking Press, 1962, p. 174.

2

Ethics and Ethos in Psychiatry: Historical Patterns and Conceptual Changes

William J. Winslade, Ph.D., J.D.

INTRODUCTION

Psychiatry is a field of human endeavor as well as a body of theory, and as such its practice is shaped and directed by the human and societal values of its practitioners. These values fall primarily into two categories: ethics and ethos. By *ethics,* I mean certain assumptions, practices and values that have directed the development of psychiatry in the 19th and 20th centuries. By *ethos,* I mean the philosophical moods—a mixture of beliefs, intentions, motives, theories and ideals—that shape the social background of psychiatric practice. By looking at certain features of the development of psychiatry, I have sought to make explicit how historical patterns in psychiatric treatment are related to shifts in the ethics and ethos of the mental health profession and the society. The history of the changes that have occurred in the mental health professional-patient relationship illustrates these

23

shifts in ethics and ethos particularly well. Because the historical patterns examined in this chapter are complex, it is difficult to make meaningful generalizations about them. The schematic outline presented in Table 1 may be of help as a guide. For example, it may be useful to scan the schematic outline horizontally for clues as to specific changes falling under a general conceptual structure.

The schematic outline can also be viewed vertically to focus attention on three main periods of development in American psychiatric practice: the Custodial period (1870-1930), the Therapeutic period (1930-1950), and the Health Systems period (1950-1980). These periods are not simply sequential lines of development; they overlap and have dominant themes that intermingle as one period gives way to the next. In each period, one or two themes are dominant, but as time passes, these themes are subordinated to others without being entirely lost. Because each period builds upon the theses of the earlier period, the pattern becomes increasingly complex. Thus, the Health Systems period includes both custodial and therapeutic variations.

In this essay, I do not advance a single thesis nor a set of interdependent propositions. My primary aim is to describe key developments. Along the way I make some assertions that point, if rather cryptically, toward explanations of the meaning and justifications of the changes that have occurred. For example, the discretionary authority of psychiatrists has shifted in both its scope and its source of justification. This shift partially results from changes in the methods of delivery of mental health care, the types of treatment offered, the interprofessional relationships between psychiatrists and other mental health professionals, the intraprofessional relationships in psychiatry, ethical shifts and legal developments. To unravel the explanations and to assess the justifications for these changes would require a more ambitious project than the survey presented here. A similar point can be made about the complex set of factors that have contributed to changes in patient status with respect to patients' rights and other key topics.

Nonetheless, certain trends have begun to take more definite

TABLE 1

Ethics in Psychiatry: Historical Patterns and Conceptual Changes

	CUSTODIAL PERIOD 1870-1930	THERAPEUTIC PERIOD 1930-1950	HEALTH SYSTEMS PERIOD 1950-present
PSYCHIATRIC TREATMENT			
ETIOLOGY	Physical and biological	Psychological and social	Biopsychosocial
TREATMENT PERSONNEL	Only physicians	Physicians, allied professionals and behavioral scientists	Treatment network — all patient contact with physician as coordinator
FORMS OF THERAPY	Therapeutic nihilism Controlled environment	Psychological Organic Drugs Psychosocial	Biopsychosocial Psychopharmacological Eclectic Systems approach
PROGNOSIS	Probably incurable	Selective responders	Uncertain outcomes and limited success
EVOLUTION OF THE MENTAL HOSPITAL	Growth in number and size of state mental hospitals as long-term facility	Transitional facilities Deinstitutionalization	Community psychiatry Least drastic alternative
TREATMENT GOALS	Control through custody	Cure with cooperation Self-actualization through insight	Relief with consent Limited by cost-effectiveness
PHILOSOPHICAL MOODS			
PSYCHIATRY	Maintenance	Intervention	Liberation and cost-effectiveness
ETHICS	Naturalism Utilitarianism Hegelian idealism	Intuitionism Pragmatism Positivism	Personal autonomy Utilitarianism Foundation of ethics uncertain
PUBLIC POLICY	State obligation (*parens patriae*)	Professional dominance and personal needs	State regulation and personal rights

TABLE 1 (*continued*)

	CUSTODIAL PERIOD 1870-1930	THERAPEUTIC PERIOD 1930-1950	HEALTH SYSTEMS PERIOD 1950-present
PROFESSIONAL STANCE			
AUTHORITY TO ACT	Political power and professional monopoly	Scientific knowledge and professional dominance	Interprofessional tensions
PROFESSIONAL RIGHTS	Decision	Discretion Prescription	Patient consent Negotiation, mutuality
PROFESSIONAL RESPONSIBILITIES	Protect patients from society and society from patients	Satisfy medical needs of individual patients; Study mental illness scientifically	Identify treatment alternatives and make recommendations
PATIENT STATUS			
COMPETENCE	Presumed incompetence (madness, lunacy)	Potential competence but impaired capacity (disease, illness and neurosis)	Presumed competence unless proven incompetent (behavioral tests)
NEEDS	Satisfaction of basic needs and segregation from society	Individualized treatment	Rehabilitation and integration into society
RIGHTS	To "custody"	Imposition of treatment	Choice of treatment, including right to refuse
RESPONSIBILITIES	To "behave"	To cooperate with treatment	To participate in decisions about treatment

shape. Psychiatric treatment has become more complex and less certain; it is ostensibly more scientific but also more controversial. Critics both inside and outside the medical and mental health community have sought to hold psychiatrists accountable. Internal critics typically emphasize scientific matters, and external critics stress ethical, legal and political considerations.

Philosophical moods have become less easy to characterize in a culture that is rapidly changing, increasingly fragmented and lacking in consensus about assumptions or aspirations. It is clear, however, that the growing influence of law on psychiatric practice has forced a shift from attention to substance to attention to procedure in setting treatment goals, establishing ethical standards and formulating public policy. It remains to be seen whether the recent increased interest in ethics will merely reflect legal developments or lead the way toward better psychiatric practices.

Changes in the relationships between psychiatrists and patients exemplify the developments in psychiatric treatment and the shifts in philosophical moods. The role of professionals has become more carefully and narrowly defined as the rights of patients have been more explicitly formulated and implemented. At the same time, the power and prestige of professionals has diminished only slightly, and perhaps more in the eyes of professionals themselves than in those of their patients. What is clear is that roles, rules and responsibilities are in transition.

In the face of these complex and difficult issues, I have not approached this essay strictly as a matter of historical research nor merely as a matter of conceptual analysis. I have used historical clues and conceptual outlines to try to create a framework for clarifying and understanding psychiatric treatment and philosophical moods in the context of the psychiatrist-patient relationship. My approach reflects my professional training as a philosopher, lawyer and psychoanalyst: I look for patterns of meaning. These patterns might be called "philosophers' history": a rational reconstruction that involves "assembling reminders for a particular purpose" (1). The particular purpose in this essay is to get our bearings in a journey that has largely been unguided.

By doing this, I hope we will be able to see the past and present in a new and illuminating way (2) leading to a more comprehensive analysis of the ethical and cultural dimensions of psychiatry.

NINETEENTH CENTURY BACKGROUND

Before turning to an elaboration of the schematic outline, it may be helpful to look at the treatment of the mentally ill in the 19th century (3). Trends in the early and mid-19th century adumbrated the Custodial, Therapeutic and Health System periods of the late 19th and 20th centuries. These trends include the emergence of the asylum, the cult of curability and certain reform movements.

Although some publicly supported mental hospitals were already in existence (4), it was not until 1828 that Horace Mann first argued that the government had an obligation to provide care for the mentally ill. Thirty-seven years later, the first law was passed in New York declaring the state's responsibility for the care of all "pauper insane." However, this law was largely ineffective, and 35 more years passed (1890) before a truly effective state law was enacted requiring all insane persons in almshouses, jails, etc., to be transferred to state hospitals and asylums as quickly as accommodations could be made ready.

This law resulted from long years of work by numerous reformers including, most prominently, Dorothea Linde Dix. Although some private facilities existed in the early part of the century, these were available only to those with financial means. Pauper lunatics were sent to almshouses in the few places where such facilities existed and, where they did not, pauper lunatics were either jailed or publicly auctioned to whoever was willing to accept the smallest amount of money for their upkeep. The appalling conditions in which pauper lunatics existed—be they in almshouses, jails, or auctioned servitude—were made public by reformers who were moved by humanitarian considerations.

Although insanity (a catchall term) had previously been considered totally incurable, the reform movement, which addressed itself primarily to decent housing, coincided with new ideas about the curability of mental illness. From about 1830-1887, popular opinion as well as much medical opinion held that mental illness was as curable as physical illness. This belief was fostered by numerous reports which manipulated and falsified statistics about cures. It was not until 1887 that the claims of the so-called cult of curability were destroyed. The resulting backlash of medical and popular opinion at that time—a return to the belief that "once insane, always insane"—meshed temporally with the widespread establishment of public asylums. These asylums initially provided more humanitarian housing, at least relative to earlier conditions. However, since there was no belief in the likelihood of cure or even of much improvement, institutionalization of the mentally ill became an end in itself.

Psychiatric theory at mid-19th century was still very limited. In the popular mind, phrenology dominated most ideas about brain function; theological ideas about the relation between sin and madness were common; diagnosis or classification of insanity by physicians was basically idiosyncratic. Some in medicine asserted that mental illness was not psychic in origin, but rather was purely physical and ultimately understandable. As Kirkbride stated in 1854, "it should never be forgotten that every individual who has a brain is liable to insanity, precisely as everyone who has lungs is liable to pneumonia" (5). But even as this idea began to take hold, it was still believed that all insane should receive the same treatment.

For the last half of the 19th century, the major treatment controversy revolved around the use of mechanical restraints. The abolition of such restraints was much more common in Europe than in the United States, despite the influence of Judge Schreber's father. Deutsch summarizes the American position as follows:

> The patients in European institutions, accustomed as they were to unquestioned acceptance of authority, might willingly submit to "moral" restraint, but not you liberty loving Americans who, sane or insane, would never agree placidly to the imposition of authority by an individual, and hence could be restrained only by mechanical means (6).

By the late 1860s, governmental centralization of welfare administration was a clearly discernible trend. In the newly-established asylums, patients were divided into two groups: curables and incurables. The problem was that there was no agreement about how to tell who belonged in which group other than by the time they had spent in the asylum. For the incurables, no treatment was necessary. For the curables, no treatment other than time, restraints and some degree of decent care was available. But both the responsibility and the power to care for the mentally ill were firmly in the hands of those who administered the asylums.

THE CUSTODIAL PERIOD, 1870-1930

Philosophical Moods

Psychiatry. In the Custodial period, professionals and the general public believed that those mentally ill persons unable to care for themselves should be cared for at public expense. Some felt that the state had an obligation to provide them with basic needs—food, clothing and shelter. Others believed that benevolence, even if not a duty, was an appropriate response to the mentally ill. Still others saw the segregation of the mentally ill from the rest of society as convenient and desirable for society. For different reasons, therefore, it was agreed that the mentally ill needed at least minimum maintenance. As a result, many mentally ill persons, especially those with chronic and severe disabilities, rejected by or without families, became wards of the state.

Minimum maintenance was all that needed to be provided and was all that was provided; indeed, as more and more patients entered hospitals and few were discharged, it was all that *could* be provided. Hospitals were remote, often located in rural settings. This physical isolation reflected society's view of the mentally ill who, out of mind, were best kept out of sight. Treatment was crude if it existed at all. Facilities were crowded, barren and inadequate. Patients were unkempt and apathetic; they engaged in few activities or social interaction, even at mealtimes. The poorly paid and usually untrained staff functioned as watchdogs over patients who were seen as a kind of subhuman species. The efforts of those compassionate reformers who worked to create the state mental hospital system had resulted, after 50 years, in what Milton Greenblatt calls "monuments of custodial stagnation and neglect" (7).

Ethics. At this time, naturalistic ethics were important and popular, as illustrated by the writings of Huxley and Spencer. Naturalists adapted Darwinism to their own purposes. Elaborating freely from the idea of the survival of the fittest, they thought of the mentally ill as unfit because they were incompetent and incurable. Naturalists believed the mentally ill should be segregated from the rest of society to prevent contamination of the human species. Some naturalists would no doubt have preferred to place them on a ship of fools and allow them to drift from port to port (8). But many persons who embraced naturalistic ethics as a theory also felt pity for such defective humans who were, after all, members of their own species, even if defective.

However, other moral forces were present in society, for example, idealism. The British philosopher T. H. Green, an idealist, has been characterized as "the apostle of state intervention in matters of social welfare" (9). For Green the state was "an embodiment of that higher self the realization of which is our moral aim." Thus, just as it was morally appropriate for the strong to protect the weak, so also was it appropriate for the state to care for the mentally disabled, according to this philosophy.

From a utilitarian point of view, in the tradition of Mill, Bentham and Sidgwick, it was apparent that segregation and minimum maintenance of the mentally ill was better for them and better for society. In calculating the costs and benefits to society as a whole, it was clear that segregation of the mentally ill was better for the patients because their needs were satisfied, and was better for society because it was protected from the discomfort and potential danger posed by lunatics. On the other hand, because the mentally ill contributed so little to society, only minimum services needed to be provided for them.

Naturalists, idealists and utilitarians could agree on one thing:

that the mentally ill were needy and dependent. Out of pity, duty or self-interest, one could justify providing some care for them. The mood of minimum maintenance thus drew upon a consensus of feelings derived from differing moral sentiments.

Public Policy. No one disputed that parents had an obligation to provide for their children. But when parents abandoned, neglected or abused their children, the state had an interest in protecting them from harm. The legal doctrine of *parens patriae,* although not new, came into full bloom in America in 1899 with the founding of the juvenile court system in Illinois, soon followed by legislation in other states. The state had an obligation to aid needy and especially potentially delinquent children (10).

Similarly, the mentally ill, often more dependent and needy than children, were sometimes abandoned, neglected or abused by their families. Moreover, both children and the mentally ill were regarded as incompetent—in fact and in law—to make important decisions for themselves. Here also the state in its *parens patriae* role should assume responsibility. This mood fueled reform movements in the 19th century and resulted in legislation establishing state hospitals. But the mentally ill—then as now—were unpopular. There was an underlying assumption that, whereas errant children could be reformed, the mentally ill could only be maintained and controlled (11). Thus the state fulfilled its obligation by providing minimal services, such as food, clothing and shelter.

Psychiatric Treatment

Etiology. The rapid growth and development of science in the 19th century in such fields as chemistry, geology and physics, gave impetus to the search for causes in medicine, including psychiatry. Mental illness was caused, most psychiatrists theorized, by physical or biological defects. Therefore, to understand mental illness, it was necessary to study the brain and the nervous system to discover underlying causes. Although research was not extensive, that which was done focused on origins rather than on cures.

The power of the deterministic hypotheses that dominated Freud's early thinking, for example, pulled research in the direction of scientific understanding of general phenomena. Little attention was paid to clinical care of particular patients. Patients were simply data for the pursuit of scientific theory.

Treatment Personnel. Only physicians were authorized to treat the mentally ill, and the treatment they provided was almost exclusively in mental hospitals. The role of the psychiatrist in this period was typically as head of a hospital. His responsibilities were to administer and to manage, not to provide treatment. Because there were no middle-level personnel, very little treatment was carried out. In theory, the hospital director could have hospital staff carry out professional directives, but in practice, the largely untrained staff were capable of little beyond physical control of their charges.

The psychiatrist stood at the top of the hierarchy, dictating the activities of the staff, often in an autocratic manner. Psychiatry as a specialty was still in its infancy, and there was little demand for psychiatrists since so few were needed to maintain authority and control in the institutions.

Forms of therapy. Redlich asserts that during the Custodial period, "there was no treatment because so-called moral treatment, essentially a humane common sense approach rather than a technology, ceased to exist when the state hospitals became large warehouses of human wrecks. Indeed there was mistreatment rather than treatment" (12). Moral treatment included a benign paternalism on the part of the physician and the caretakers and necessitated residence in an asylum, where conditions could be controlled so that the disordered moral faculties of the insane person's mind could be restored to their proper functioning. However, as the hospitals became increasingly crowded, the idea of controlling the environment was abandoned in favor of controlling the patients. Greenblatt points out that:

> . . . perhaps the worst features of hospitals prior to the 1930s were their "therapeutic" procedures, then regarded as necessary or even progressive, but now seen as punitive, restrictive,

rejecting and laced with routinization and impersonalization (13).

He goes on to describe the use of seclusion, forced tube-feeding, chemical restraint, continuous tubs, physical restraints, and wet packs. These are no longer considered by many to be appropriate forms of therapy, although debate about the therapeutic and non-therapeutic value of seclusion exists to this day.

Nonetheless, institutionalization did sometimes result in therapeutic benefits for patients. The benefits were largely a result of environmental factors, such as removal from stressful or conflictual social situations, or contacts with humane, even if not well-qualified, staff. Of course, some patients got better because their psychiatric condition was time-limited. The mental institution at least provided maintenance while the person recovered.

Prognosis. As in the early 19th century, the prognosis for most mentally ill persons was poor during the Custodial period. Their condition was believed to result from incurable biological or physical defects. The adage "once insane, always insane" prevailed. Thus, "many patients stayed for long months and even years . . . once admitted, they were forever stigmatized, even if they were fortunate enough to be discharged" (14).

Evolution of the Mental Hospital. Several factors contributed to the growth in size and number of state mental hospitals. First, the state manifested its *parens patriae* assumption of responsibility through legislation. Second, as facilities became available, patients were drawn not only from jails and poorhouses, but also from families which, for various reasons, would not or could not care for mentally disabled relatives. As the idea of sending a burdensome relative to a hospital became more acceptable in a society that was increasingly intolerant both of eccentricity and of defects, families no longer felt they had to care for mentally disabled relatives. Third, because patients remained in mental hospitals for relatively long periods of time, admissions outnumbered discharges. And fourth, once the idea of the mental hospital was concretized, it served multiple professional, political, moral and personal purposes. As a result of these factors, the original concept of a mental hospital as a small facility caring for about 250 persons was rapidly replaced by the reality of a huge fortress-like institution with as many as 10,000 patients (15).

Treatment Goals. The primary treatment goal in this period can be summarized in a phrase: control through custody. Control was manifested in increasingly restrictive ways: Institutionalization itself was control, and isolation, seclusion, sheet packs, etc. were further forms of control. Control was exercised not to cure but to reduce the opportunity for bad behavior. Because control was best achieved and maintained through custody, institutionalization was the logical result. Further, since most mentally ill persons were either incurable or would recover on their own, custodial care was believed to be appropriate and adequate. The limited horizons of psychiatric treatment were matched by the mood of minimum maintenance reflected in psychiatry, ethics and public policy.

Professional Stance

Authority to Act. There were two primary sources of authority for psychiatrists in the Custodial period: the political power of the state and professional dominance. Mental hospitals were authorized and constructed by the state; funds for construction and selection of builders were controlled, as usual, by the political patronage system. But the state was not interested in exerting much direct control over the actual operation of the institution; power was, therefore, vested largely in the hospital superintendents, who were typically psychiatrists. This process fed into psychiatrists' growing desire for professional autonomy. Backed by the imprimatur of the state, the psychiatrist-superintendent could exercise authoritarian control over the staff and patients.

Physicians were the only professionally organized and powerful group. Redlich claims that "other professions were not on the scene" (16). The small number of nurses, social workers and occupational therapists who were in the hospitals were, thus, already dominated professionally by the physicians, and their position was further weakened by the political process described above. One consequence of this structuring of authority and status was a serious quality problem. The day-to-day operation of the hospital was largely carried out by nonprofessional staff or by professionals so poorly qualified that they might as well have been nonprofessionals. Greenblatt observes that many staff members

> found themselves overwhelmed. Vacancies were frequent, recruitment difficult, job gratification limited. Many of these staff members lived in the hospital where a room was supplied free of charge, meals were taken in cafeterias, and socialization was inbred. Thus the hospital workers, too, retreated from society; often they felt ill-equipped to meet the vicissitudes of life outside, and were unmotivated, therefore, in helping the patient to adapt to the real world (17).

Professional Rights. It has already been mentioned that physicians were the only professionals authorized to treat patients, another example of the professional dominance characteristic of the Custodial period. The psychiatrist, who might spend very little time in actual patient contact, had the right to decide what treatment, if any, should be provided and whether the patient should be discharged (18). He was thus able to exercise a remarkable amount of discretion with effectively no one in a position to question his judgment or to make independent decisions.

Professional Responsibilities. The psychiatrist's responsibilities were defined in terms of protection: protecting patients from themselves and protecting society from the patients. Psychiatrists, therefore, exercised *parens patriae* power with respect to protecting the mentally ill from themselves, and police power with respect to protecting society from the mentally ill. This division of loyalties produced an ambiguous role that has continued to be problematic for some psychiatrists, especially those who have authority to hospitalize patients against their will. However, many psychiatrists readily accepted this dual role, since law and social values supported both aspects of it. The paternalistic role was compatible with the emergence of the physician as a professionally powerful and dominant force in society. The primary task for the psychiatrist was to *control* the patients, and custody was seen as the best means for establishing control. Anything else done for patients—treatment, rehabilitation, cure or discharge— had to be achieved within the framework of custodial control.

Patient Status

Competence. From a legal and moral standpoint, mental patients were presumed incompetent for practically all purposes. Madness or lunacy was viewed not only as a physical or biological defect, but also as a defect that diminished the human status of the patient. As the mentally ill were generally believed to be incurable, their illness was perceived as a permanent state that effectively rendered them incompetent not because their judgment was diminished but because they were something less than or dif- ferent from other humans. The mentally ill person was, as Green- blatt says, forever stigmatized. Therefore mental patients could be treated as subhumans: warehoused, herded and often ex- ploited. For example:

> showers and bathing were carried out on a mass basis with- out regard for privacy. Toilet functions were non-private and toilet seats were often lacking. Poverty, empty hours and lack of personal attention made the individual an inmate or a number rather than a true patient who received medical and psychiatric diagnosis and treatment. He was far from a true citizen or vital member of any social group (19).

Needs. Social attitudes about Blacks and slavery as well as the theories of Social Darwinism encouraged the notion that some groups of human beings could be considered different in both degree and kind from other humans. Applied to mental patients, this thinking suggested that they were less human than other people. Food, clothing and shelter at the barest levels were suffi- cient; spiritual needs—socialization, education, culture—were be- lieved to be beyond their capacity or desire. Rather than parti- cipating in society, they required, perhaps preferred, segregation

from society. This isolationist thinking tended to reduce further
the status of mentally ill persons; for, like many prisoners and
slaves, they tended to adapt their needs to what was available
to them. The belief, during the Custodial period, that the needs
of the mentally ill were minimal became a self-fulfilling presumption.

Rights. Little if any attention was given to individual rights of
mental patients. Although society might have a duty of benevolence to those in need, the needy had no *a priori right* to benevolence. It was in every sense more blessed to give than to receive.
The most explicitly expressed theme of the time was the general
duty of the state to assist the needy. The concept of individual
rights or personal rights had not been articulated either in social
ethics or in law. One might even say that the primary right of the
mentally ill, like that of dependent and delinquent children, was
the right to custody: to be taken care of and to be controlled.

Responsibilities. Because the mentally ill were classified as
incompetent, it may seem inappropriate to speak of their responsibilities. Nevertheless, it was implied that the mentally ill had a
responsibility to behave cooperatively—to cause no disruptions,
to make no demands, to stay out of trouble. The so-called therapies described previously were frequently used as punishments
for misbehavior, to keep the difficult patients in line. In general,
if mental patients remained passive and compliant, they were left
alone and perhaps discharged.

THE THERAPEUTIC PERIOD, 1930-1950

Philosophical Moods

Psychiatry. At the beginning of the 20th century, the mood in
psychiatry began to shift from maintenance to intervention. The
maintenance mentality still existed, but the discovery of new and
sometimes radical forms of therapy held out the promise that at
least some previously unreachable patients might be helped by
active treatment (20), even though others could still only be
maintained. Thus, selective intervention, a much more optimis-

tic mood, began to gain ground. As we shall see, several factors contributed to this new mood.

Lack of restriction on scientific experimentation gave impetus to psychiatric research and also to new methods of clinical treatment. The expansion of psychiatry as a profession as well as the growth of other mental health professions—psychology, social work and nursing—created a supply of professionals prepared to meet and even stimulate a demand for mental health services. The new professionals, encouraged by the growth of the social sciences, theorized that social factors were responsible for mental illness and thus, in order to help the mentally ill, their environment must be reshaped. The image of the mental hospital was changed from a warehouse to a community life, which also contributed to the new mood of intervention. A less pessimistic and deterministic attitude toward the mentally ill began to emerge. The concept of mental illness itself was expanded to include less severe and more treatable forms of mental disorder in addition to psychosis; treatment of severe mental illness, previously dismissed as impossible, was seen as potentially fruitful in individual cases.

Ethics. During the Therapeutic period, several philosophical movements contributed to value changes that were particularly relevant to psychiatry. Naturalistic ethics, though still a popular attitude, had come under considerable attack from several groups. The intuitionists, such as G. E. Moore and H. A. Pritchard, believed that what was good or right could not be learned from science or evolution. They believed that values were independent of nature and that to try to derive values from facts was fallacious. Instead, the intuitionists believed a value was, as Justice Potter Stewart later said of obscenity, something you know when you see it. Although intuitionism is primarily of interest to professional philosophers, it related to a characteristic attitude in the early 20th century, namely, that humans are not merely slaves of nature, but have a capacity to experience and appreciate intrinsic values. This attitude was also consistent with the view that at least some persons have the capacity to perceive what is good and right, not only for themselves but also for others. As we shall see, professionals and scientists riding on the crest of scientific success in our credentialed society designated themselves as the possessors of such enlightened vision.

Another philosophical movement, in some ways at odds with intuitionism, also supported the view that values are nonnatural properties. This was the logical positivist movement that originated with the Vienna Circle but quickly gained adherents in America where science had become such a dominant social force. The logical positivists believed that the only meaningful statements were those that could be empirically verified. All other claims, such as statements about ethics or other values, were matters of emotion and feeling that were inherently unverifiable.

The positivists tended to glorify the pursuit of scientific knowledge; the task of philosophers was to purify scientific language. By decreeing that only scientists could make truly meaningful statements, the positivists elevated science to a position of authority over other fields. In a sense, the message of the positivists was that only scientists knew what they were talking about. This attitude gave backing to the notion that professional scientists were in a better position than anyone else not only to discover what was true or false, but also to know what was best. Although this implicit message is a non sequitur, the prestige and power of science prevailed over mere logic, especially in a society inebriated with the power of science and technology to change the course of nature. Thus the spirit of positivist theory reinforced the practice of scientific interventionism. Because psychiatry had scientific status, interventionism meshed well with psychiatry's professional dominance, which was derived from political power, psychological authority and the scientific base of medicine.

A third philosophical movement characteristic of American culture was the pragmatism of William James and John Dewey. Pragmatism endorsed both scientific knowledge and the experimental attitude as it blended with typically American utilitarian sentiments: Truth is what works. Trial and error was recognized to be a necessary stage in the development of scientific knowledge. Pragmatism was oriented toward problem-solving, practical solutions and, above all, toward flexibility and openness to new methods, revised goals and structural changes. The pragmatic mood differed from positivism in that it was less interested in verification than in implementation, but shared with positivism the belief that scientific knowledge was a worthy goal. Where scientific knowledge was lacking, a scientific method must be adopted to seek it. Pragmatism endorsed the use of scientific intervention to control and even conquer nature, to adapt natural forces to human purposes, and to give new shape and direction to human society. It is easy to see how the pragmatic mood was compatible with the therapeutic mood in psychiatry.

Just as scientific engineering could radically alter the physical landscape, so it was believed that scientific psychiatry could alter the interiors of the mind. Thus, the scientific status of psychiatry and psychoanalysis—in contrast to psychology (viewed as a pseudoscience) or social work (viewed as a wholly pragmatic but nonscientific activity) or nursing (viewed as a subservient profession)—was elevated to a position of power and prestige. Therefore, psychiatrists as professional scientists felt justified in intervening in the treatment of the mentally ill because they knew what was best for their patients: As scientists, they had the method to verify their beliefs, and as pragmatic clinicians, they were entitled to try alternative interventions to see what worked.

Public Policy. With the doctrine of *parens patriae* fully established and firmly entrenched, there was a shift to implementation of scientifically sound treatments in the Therapeutic period. During the Custodial period, public policy had favored minimal regulation, delegating authority for all decisions about treatment to the professionals who ran the hospitals, and particularly to the psychiatrists. In the Therapeutic period, public policy remained the same: minimal regulation with professionals making treatment decisions. However, because professionals were committed to trying new forms of treatment, the policy of minimal regulation implicitly endorsed flexible treatment for individual needs as well as sometimes abusive therapeutic and research practices. Abuses were particularly common in the overcrowded, understaffed and undermanned institutions. Not until late in the Therapeutic period was there any public interest in treatment practices or conditions in these institutions, and thus no popular or political force to counter their lack of regulation. When public interest was provoked, as it was, for example, by the novel and movie *The Snake Pit,* this policy of minimal regulation was, for the first time, seriously questioned.

Psychiatric Treatment

Etiology. In addition to physical and biological causes of mental illness, psychological and social factors were now also explicitly acknowledged as causes. The emergence and growth of psychoanalysis as a general psychology, along with the expansion of pyschology as a profession, reflected this change, and helped people to accept the idea of the mentally ill person's need for treatment and the possibility of effective treatment. The classification of neurosis as a mental illness enlarged the scope of mental illness in a significant way, drawing attention to a larger population's need for treatment. Although the general public received this idea with mixed feelings, the scientific community was relatively willing to accept the idea that mental illness was not limited to the unfortunate inmates of mental hospitals, but existed in a wider population—including juvenile delinquents, criminals and malcontents—if not, at least potentially, in everyone (21).

Treatment Personnel. Whereas in the Custodial period, only physicians were authorized to treat patients, in the Therapeutic period, psychiatrists were aided by and worked in conjunction with allied professionals, principally psychologists, social workers and nurses. In addition, as Greenblatt points out, collaboration between psychiatrists and behavioral scientists was a result of "interest in social milieu as a therapeutic force." He goes on to say that:

> The alliance of psychiatry with sociology, anthropology, social psychology and behavioral science produced substantial benefits in patient care and treatment. Such factors as set, expectation, social interaction, goals, rewards, the overt and covert ideological tenets and values in each ward unit, and,

above all, the climate or atmosphere that characterized an institution were now added to this list of therapeutic variables. Scientists from humanistic fields began to see the mental hospital as a place where a career could be fashioned (22).

Forms of Therapy. During the Therapeutic period, many forms of therapy proliferated, including organic, chemical, psychological and psychosocial techniques. These well-known developments are summarized by Greenblatt as follows:

> In the 1930s with the introduction of somatic therapies, such as electric shock, insulin hypoglycemia, and lobotomy, a transformation began to take place in state mental hospitals. Electric shock gave dramatic relief to crippling depressions and involutional melancholia. Insulin-coma therapy appeared to be of benefit to schizophrenic patients, and lobotomy was reported to relieve anxious agitation in a variety of chronic "hopeless" individuals (23).

It should be added that the influence of psychoanalysis, especially in the 1930s with the influx of central European psychoanalysts to the United States, was a significant force. Redlich summarizes this development:

> Psychoanalysis held out considerable promise to explain human behavior better than other systems. As a therapeutic instrument it offered not only systematic treatment but actualization of one's potential, a diminution of conflict, particularly guilt, and an expansion of consciousness. Psychoanalytically trained psychiatrists became leaders of their profession. American psychoanalysts disregarded Freud's recommendation not to discriminate against non-medical analysts. It became, for a while at least, a medical specialty. A large number of psychiatrists sought analytic training and engaged in analytic practice. It encouraged teachers and students of psychoanalysis to address not only the headaches of living but also a great variety of human enterprises and problems. . . . (24).

Prognosis. The Therapeutic period did not repeat the excesses of the cult of curability in the 19th century, but there was a new optimism. As Greenblatt points out, the new forms of therapy led to "revolutionary new attitudes about the prognosis of patients long regarded as therapeutically recalcitrant" (25). This enthusiasm was not limited to prognoses concerning the institutionalized mentally ill. It extended to persons with adjustment problems—delinquents, criminals and other misfits—who might benefit from medical or psychological therapy, counseling, social intervention, etc. To a certain extent, there was a belief that psychiatry could cure social as well as personal ills. At this stage, the psychologizing of social action and individual conduct became commonplace (26). Later we shall see how this theoretical enthusiasm was translated into practical consequences.

Evolution of the Mental Hospital. During the Therapeutic period, significant changes in the mental hospital structure resulted primarily from two factors: introduction of new therapies promising positive results and the development of ideas about the therapeutic value of the mental health community. Electroshock, insulin hypoglycemia and lobotomy promised dramatic new possibilities for patients whose condition had long been considered hopeless. This new optimism created a revitalization of mental health workers, and psychotherapeutic techniques were used with a new interest and aggressiveness. Social scientists, who were particularly instrumental in furthering interest in developing the social environment of the hospitals for therapeutic purposes, discovered a role for themselves in the activities of the mental hospital. Increasingly, scientific research that included a humanistic viewpoint was conducted. The introduction of a new group of professionals, along with the new hope for cures or at least significant improvements for many patients, created a climate in which cooperation among workers was seen to be important. This collegial environment did much to break down the authoritarian chain of command of the Custodial period. Although psychiatrists still held primary responsibility for the care of patients, staff members themselves began to take on responsibilities for patients' treatment, rather than assuming that only the physician's or psychiatrist's direct treatment could be helpful.

Treatment Goals. Patients with acute or chronic mental illness or symptomatic complaints were now believed to have potentially favorable prognoses. For these patients, a trial-and-error approach to selecting a form of therapy was recommended. Clinical care was approached with a scientific attitude and in a pragmatic spirit. It was hoped that at least some responsive individuals could be successfully treated, even if the ills of society could only be diagnosed but not cured. The key to cure was the capacity and willingness of the patient to cooperate with the treatment.

Similarly, the treatment goal for the neurotic patient was self-actualization through insight. The patient in psychotherapy or psychoanalysis was expected to accept the recommendations of the therapist concerning the nature and course of treatment. The therapist established the rules and a compliant patient followed them. If the patient cooperated by accepting transference, dependence and therapeutic authority, there was the prospect of being successfully or fully analyzed.

Professional Stance

Authority to Act. The authority of psychiatrists during the Therapeutic period expanded from political power and professional dominance based on professional prestige to include professional dominance based on alleged scientific knowledge. Other mental health professionals were still not well-organized and established; they were invited to collaborate with psychiatrists as long as they respected the hierarchical structure of medical authority. In addition to the transference-based authority of physicians (27), the legitimacy of science gave psychiatrists an unusually powerful position, at least with respect to treatment of the mentally ill. Even if the general public remained suspicious and fearful about the imperialistic tendencies of psychiatry during this period, psychiatrists' authority to treat the mentally ill was not seriously challenged. For example, Redlich points out that:

> The Second World War changed the world and had a major impact on American psychiatry. Two notable events took place. The first was the feat of American psychiatrists to

keep one million young men from being drafted for psychiatric reasons, and later, to discharge almost two millions with
psychiatric diagnoses. The generals were impressed as David
Musto put it. It never became clear whether the USA won
the war because of this or in spite of it! The military and
civilian leadership as well as the psychiatrists who served
in the armed forces during the war were also impressed with
the achievements of psychotherapy with combat troops.
There was hope that similar results could be achieved with
civilian populations (28).

and:

The post war period was a period of remarkable growth of
private practice, first of psychiatry, later of clinical psychology and social work, and to a lesser extent of nursing.
The patients of such practice were mostly neurotic and not
psychotics and sociopaths; the mentally deficient was out of
"psychiatry's sight and interest." The practice of "dynamic"
psychotherapy (or shouldn't it be called psychoeducation?)
became the common ground but also the bone of contention
of the professions (29).

Professional Rights. As a result of this considerable authority
to act, psychiatrists during the Therapeutic period had significant
discretionary powers. They exercised discretion with respect to
all medical and scientific matters concerning their patients—diagnosis, forms of treatment, patient interaction with other professionals, and even intervention into other aspects of a patient's
life. Psychiatrists were seen as experts not only in matters of
scientific knowledge, but also in problems of living. Although we
all know that Szasz overstates his case, his central thesis about the
ways that psychiatrists have been invited to play the role and have
accepted the part of experts on the problems of living has a
fundamental truth to it. However, Szasz does not adequately
acknowledge the extent to which psychiatrists have been pushed
into this role by the demands of a troubled society. The decline
of traditional sources of authority and the tremendous progress
made in psychiatry by the mid-20th century gave psychiatry a new
prominence and power. During the Therapeutic period, psychia-

trists enjoyed more discretion and less challenge than they ever had before or are likely to have again.

By the end of the 1950s, psychiatrists were expected to prescribe a cure—pills, psychotherapy, organic treatment—for individual and social ills. If a prescription was made, it was presumed that it would be followed. Psychiatrists did not ask patients what they wanted or felt they needed; rather patients were told what to do. Similarly, psychiatrists often served as consultants to schools, courts and policy makers. The initial impact of psychiatry on criminal law of insanity through the ill-fated *Durham* rule illustrates this trend. It was assumed that psychiatric expertise could be used to unravel the mysteries of human nature and be utilized to control human conduct.

Professional Responsibilities. The primary responsibility of the psychiatrist during the Therapeutic period was to satisfy the individual medical needs of his/her patients. The available resources were considerable: better trained allied professionals, new forms of therapy, more positive prognoses for many patients and revitalized mental hospitals. In addition, the scientific status and discretionary authority of the psychiatrist were generally accepted, if not by a suspicious public, at least by many persons in positions of power. It was felt that psychiatrists could and would help their patients by designing individualized treatment plans for each one of them. In this way, all available resources would be brought to bear concretely on the clinical care of particular patients.

In view of a deferential public and a positive political attitude toward psychiatry in this period, it is not surprising that ample funds were available to permit a pragmatic approach to clinical care to be supplanted by a more rigorously scientific approach to the problems of mental illness. Redlich points out that:

> For psychiatry the most significant event of the post war years was the establishment of the National Institutes of Health, one of them the National Institute of Mental Health. Since its inception it has played a very important role in the development of research in psychiatry and its basic biological and psychological and social sciences. Another powerful

federal agency, the Veterans Administration, not only provided good care for the returning soldier, but added significantly to the national research effort. The research budget of the National Institute of Mental Health rose rapidly, enabling scientists in psychiatry and its basic sciences to work under conditions promoting excellence. It also became possible to train a cadre of young clinical and basic scientists, establishing a leadership position of American mental health research in the world (30).

This initiated the movement toward seeing psychiatry as a science of mental health as well as a science of mental illness. Psychiatrists began to perceive their responsibilities as going beyond the care of the individual patient to prescribing regimens and remedies—in education, politics, law and culture—for the prevention of mental illness and the preservation of mental health.

Patient Status

Competence. In the Therapeutic period, in contrast to the Custodial period, mental illness was perceived to be less an irreparable defect than a potentially curable illness or disease. Mentally ill persons were seen as not completely competent but not permanently incompetent. The goal was to restore them, if not to full competence, at least to their maximum functional level. In a sense, this period reflects the mood of self-realization articulated earlier by philosophers such as F. H. Bradley and T. M. Green. All persons should be permitted to realize their capacities to the fullest possible degree. This was reinforced by the influence of psychoanalysis as a form of therapy leading to self-development—a "second education" as Freud put it.

Needs. Accordingly, the individual needs of all persons must be identified in order to help them realize their own unique capacities. A similar rhetoric was widely promulgated in the juvenile justice system for dealing with delinquent and dependent children. In psychiatry, this worthy ideal was extremely difficult to achieve for a variety of reasons. Psychoanalysis, the therapeutic method most suited to intense individualized treatment, was expensive, lengthy and had uncertain results. The effectiveness of other forms of therapy, such as behavior modification and drug treatment, in general, had not been verified. The effectiveness of any form of therapy in a particular case could be determined only after trial and error; this included risking side effects and negative consequences. Although clinical experimentation might be permissible as a last resort with patients recalcitrant to treatment, it was uncertain whether private and public outpatients should be subjected to unproven therapeutic procedures. Psychiatry aspired to science but operated as well-intentioned pragmatism. Individualized treatment was desirable but very difficult to achieve. Psychoanalysts, following Freud's shift from initial optimism about symptomatic relief to doubts about the possibility of characterological cures, began to pull back just as other mental health professionals began to make enticing promises. Of course, many psychiatrists who were also psychoanalysts merely lost their enthusiasm for analysis, not their conviction that mental illness was curable or at least controllable.

Rights. Because the outlook for mental health care was promising, patients had a right to be treated. This required increased political and economic support for psychiatric training, research and clinical care. The budget of NIMH was enlarged. Politicians were urged to pass laws not only to benefit voluntary patients who sought treatment, but also to require mentally ill persons to be treated, if necessary, against their will. If the mentally ill did not recognize their own needs, psychiatrists should have the power to do it for them. Thus many states passed involuntary commitment laws based upon the professional clinical judgment of a psychiatrist.

Responsibilities. The patient, to be cured, had to cooperate with treatment. It was not enough for the patient to be the passive recipient of mental health care. Patients had to be educated, had to be taught that treatment was in their best interests. When the patient recognized that he/she was mentally ill—had emotional problems—then the patient was prepared to be cured. To deny mental illness was itself a symptom of the condition.

THE HEALTH SYSTEMS PERIOD (1950-1980)

Philosophical Moods

Psychiatry. In the last 30 years, the mood in psychiatry has been an unstable mixture of the ideal of liberation and the reality of cost-effectiveness. The ideal of liberation has been partially achieved with the help of various drugs which relieve some of the most disabling symptoms of mental illness. (Many afflicted persons can function, with at least some success, outside an institutional setting. Drugs can, of course, also be used within institutional settings to control mental disorders enough to permit other forms of therapy to be used conjointly.)

However, it is clear that drugs are neither necessary nor sufficient for liberation from mental disorder. Psychopharmacology does partially answer the search for a scientific and medical solution to mental illness, but it is well-known that some conditions and some persons, unresponsive to medication, do respond to other forms of treatment, such as psychotherapy or behavior modification. Thus, drugs are not always necessary. They are also not always sufficient for liberation because, though they may provide relief for some symptoms, they do not necessarily cure the problem. Drugs are only instruments for treatment that can be used, as we all know, for good or evil. The overuse of drugs as a means of control and as a substitute for individualized care is an all-too-familiar phenomenon. Finally, even when drugs have been effectively used to enable mentally ill persons to be released from inpatient treatment, subsequent outpatient care has not always been adequate. As a result, many patients require repeated hospitalizations to stabilize their condition. Nevertheless, it is fair to say that liberation with the aid of drugs has been one dominant theme in contemporary psychiatry.

With drug treatment, relief of certain symptoms can be achieved rather rapidly in contrast to long-term psychotherapy or psychoanalysis. This is important because cost-effectiveness puts a premium on time needed for treatment, especially in high-overhead institutional settings. Liberation from mental illness should not, of course, be confused with release from a hospital or termination of treatment. But both patients and professionals, anxious to reduce costs, may be satisfied with fewer emotional benefits if the alternative is substantially more costly.

Cost-effectiveness is also compatible with the American impatience with anything that cannot, at least in theory, be done quickly. The proliferations of instant cures and "quickie" therapies is a response to this demand. A similar attitude is reflected in federal and state support for mental health care. Effectiveness is measured in terms of decreased length of hospitalization or decreased frequency of outpatient visits. This does decrease short-term economic costs, even if the long-term psychological costs are not reduced but actually increased, especially if one takes into account repeated hospitalizations. What is lost in this process is the commitment to the ideal of individualized treatment. Even if it was rarely achieved in the Therapeutic period, it was a worthy goal. It has been replaced by the Medicare mentality that measures cure in quantitative rather than in qualitative terms.

There are other reasons why psychopharmacology is a particularly attractive tool for psychiatrists. It brings psychiatry more directly into the mainstream of science and medicine, and also bolsters a waning professional dominance: Only physicians can prescribe drugs (31). Moreover, the use of drugs is compatible with earlier philosophical moods in psychiatry. Drugs are often, if not always appropriately, used for *control* of the mentally ill. And they are a concrete form of *intervention* that usually have a discernible effect. Thus, even psychiatrists who do not view drugs as vehicles for liberation can use them without much fear of criticism. However, an anti-drug movement is growing, in legal circles as well as in some health-related disciplines.

Ethics. As Redlich and Mollica (32) point out, there has been an impressive new interest in professional ethics, and particularly in medical ethics, during the last 10 years. The moral dimensions of psychiatric care in particular have just begun to receive adequate attention. But unlike previous periods when the presence of philosophy was felt through philosophical movements, it has recently been most evident through conflicting ethical orientations. The recurrent theme in much current literature on this topic is the tension between person-oriented and social benefit-oriented ethics. These themes were articulated in 1970 by Paul Ramsey in *The Patient as Person* (33). They continue to echo. Person-oriented ethics has its philosophical roots in both Kantian philosophy and 19th century liberalism, but the most important additional support comes from American law. The concern about personal autonomy in ethics could never have become such a potent political force were it not that American law places such a strong emphasis on personal rights (e.g., in criminal law, protections for persons accused of crimes; in civil law, remedies in torts for persons harmed by negligence, as in medical malpractice).

On the other hand, the strong utilitarian trends in American culture emphasizing a cost-benefit approach to public policy have also played an important role in shaping ethical attitudes. A particularly striking example is found in the attitudes of researchers and scientists toward human subject research. It is widely felt that science requires the participation of human subjects to determine whether new therapies are more effective than old ones. The significant progress that has been made in studying the effectiveness of drugs for the treatment of mental illness could never have been accomplished without the administration of such drugs to mental patients, usually institutionalized patients. From a utilitarian point of view, this is a justifiable process. However, person-oriented ethicists tend to be critical of it.

It has become clear that there is a tension between the moral demands of a person-oriented approach to ethics and those of a utilitarian approach in the context of scientific research. Much of the recent work of the National Commission for the Protection of Human Subjects of Biomedical and Behavioral Research revolved around this tension, and the Commission's reports attempt to find ways to accommodate both ethical approaches in formulating recommendations for public policy. Attorneys favor person-oriented ethics, and research scientists lean toward utilitarian ethics, with philosophers lining up on both sides. Psychiatrists also seem to divide along the lines of patient-oriented and public health-oriented care, the former being more compatible with ethics of personal autonomy and the latter with ethics of social benefit. Psychiatrists in private practice typically fall into the first group, and institution-based psychiatrists are more commonly aligned with the second group.

What has emerged is an increasing awareness of the presence of ethical issues and the need to attend to them. In their superb article, "Overview: Ethical Issues in Contemporary Psychiatry," Redlich and Mollica point out that not only physicians but also philosophers, theologians, social and behavioral scientists, psychoanalysts and lawyers have become concerned with ethics (32). With so many different disciplines and professions attempting to grapple with the issues, it is not surprising that there is conflict, competition and controversy. Indeed, many contemporary discussions of ethical dilemmas seem unresolvable and interminable. The cause of this, in addition to reasoning based on differing assumptions, is that the foundations of ethics themselves are uncertain and elusive. In a particularly suggestive article, the philosopher Alasdair McIntyre attempts to explain "The Frustrating Search for the Foundation of Ethics." His central thesis is that:

> Our society stands at the meeting-point of a number of different histories, each of them the bearer of a highly particular kind of moral tradition, each of those traditions to some large degree mutilated and fragmented by its encounter with the others. The institutions of the American Polity, with their appeal to abstract universality, and to consensus, are in fact a place of encounter for rival and incompatible outlooks to a degree that the consensus itself requires should not be acknowledged. The image of the American is a mask that, because it must be worn by blacks, Indians, Japanese and Swedes, by Irish Catholics, New England Puritans, German Lutherans and rootless secularists, can fit no face very well. It is small wonder that the confusions of pluralism are articulated at the level of moral argument in the forms of a mishmash of conceptual fragments (34).

The conceptual fragmentation of which McIntyre speaks is certainly mirrored in the history of American philosophy in the past century. The proliferation of movements, moods, doctrines and dogmas is at least astonishing if not overwhelming. Not only have philosophers disagreed since the time of Plato about what philosophy is, but disagreement about assumptions, methods and conclusions has been elevated to a virtue *par excellence* in philosophy. This is especially true in the history of ethics and is clearly illustrated by Redlich and Mollica's review article.

Public Policy. During the Health Systems period, the most significant change in public policy with respect to psychiatry has been the increasing amount of state regulation, not only of funding and licensing, but of psychiatric treatment itself. The era of professional dominance has been replaced by the era of professional accountability. This shift has been felt in many areas of psychiatric practice—involuntary commitment, the right to treatment, the right to release, expert testimony, the use of medication, etc. Similarly, psychiatric research has been subject to increasing regulation by institutional review boards as well as by federal and state statutes and regulations. Although debate about the desirability and consequences of increased governmental regulation has not resulted in consensus, it is generally agreed that regulation will significantly shape the patterns of psychiatric care in the last segment of the 20th century.

Public policy emphasis has shifted from the Therapeutic period's concern about personal *needs* of patients (to which health professionals are most sensitive) to the Health Systems period's concern about the personal *rights* of patients (to which lawyers are most attuned). This may be an aspect of a general legal trend toward recognition of the personal rights of minority groups who have suffered from political discrimination. The mentally ill as a class have suffered from political discrimination. They suffer not only from their handicaps, but also from their vulnerability to neglect and exploitation and their relative lack of political power compared to racial and ethnic minorities. Thus, it is only recently that the mentally handicapped, in contrast to the better organized developmentally disabled, have begun to acquire political prominence. Federal legislation is currently being considered by the Senate Health Committee to enact a mental patient's Bill of Rights that would reinforce the rhetoric, even if not the reality, of this trend toward emphasizing rights rather than needs.

Psychiatric Treatment

Etiology. In the Custodial period, physical and biological factors were thought to cause mental illness; in the Therapeutic period, psychological and social factors were given prominence. In the Health Systems period, it is recognized that all such factors can contribute to mental illness. There is less interest in identifying single factors and more concern with assessing the relative significance of the multiple factors that may contribute to mental illness. Thus, the term *biopsychosocial* is used to refer to the cluster of causes of mental illness that must be examined in order to determine the importance of each factor for each case.

Interest in the causation of mental illness has waned as treatment has become more oriented toward relief of symptoms, regardless of their etiology. Psychiatric researchers continue to seek the causes of mental illness, but psychiatric clinicians tend to assume multiple causation and often use conjunctive therapies— medication, individual and group therapy, rehabilitation, etc. Especially in difficult cases of mixed diagnosis, psychiatric treatment is often based on a pragmatic approach—try it and see if it works. This pragmatic approach may be particularly characteristic of those engaged in therapeutic research, where there is a blending of the researcher/clinician roles. This kind of research is very difficult to control, because it requires such a high level of clinical judgment in the absence of reliable information about standard treatments.

Treatment Personnel. The expansion of treatment personnel during the Therapeutic period to include health professionals other than psychiatrists has led to a restructuring of mental health services. In institutionalized mental health care, all members of the treatment team now have patient contact. This has led to interprofessional competition about treatment and decision-making, although the psychiatrist usually serves as the coordinator of the team as well as the treating physician. To some extent, this arrangement reflects an attempt by psychiatrists to retain their professional dominance while relinquishing some control over patient care.

In noninstitutionalized mental health, psychiatrists no longer dominate the field of psychotherapy. Not only must psychiatrists compete with traditional mental health professionals, but also with the many fringe and alternative therapies which have gained adherents. In addition, self-help and peer counseling have developed to fill a need that is not being met by psychiatrists.

Forms of Therapy. Forms of therapy have proliferated during the Health Systems period. Psychiatrists, along with other mental health professionals, offer a wide range of therapies including individual and group psychotherapy from various orientations, family therapy, marital therapy, psychoanalysis, and varieties of eccentric and radical therapies that, in Los Angeles at least, are too numerous to mention. The distinctive form of therapy that psychiatrists can offer is psychopharmacological, the combined use of drugs and other forms of therapy. In addition to drugs that provide sedation, the more sophisticated medications include agents to modify pyschosis; e.g., depression, mania, and thought disorders of various kinds. Brain chemistry has provided clues to both the causes and potential cures for mental illness, and the drug revolution has given psychiatric research new momentum.

Prognosis. Despite renewed enthusiasm for psychotropic drugs (35), the prognosis for most mentally ill individuals remains uncertain. The absence of adequately documented outcome studies of the various forms of therapy, including drugs, hampers the making of reliable prognoses. Although drugs have enabled many mentally ill persons to live outside institutional settings, the relief has often been palliative rather than curative. Short-term relief has not always led to long-term recovery. Many chronically mentally ill individuals, released from institutions, have been housed in urban ghettos. Even if medication has provided some relief, psychosocial services for the noninstitutionalized mentally ill have been inadequate. Thus only limited success has been achieved.

Evolution of the Mental Hospital. The number of patients in mental hospitals has now dramatically decreased as a result, in large part, of anti-psychotic medications. The use of drugs in mental hospitals has also changed the atmosphere for those who remain institutionalized. For many patients who have been released from hospitals, the ideal form of treatment includes outpatient care and related community services. The community psychiatry movement of the 1960s sought to satisfy the needs of patients who earlier would have remained hospitalized. Lack of long-term funding has, however, undermined large-scale development of community psychiatry. Moreover, promises that community psychiatry would be less expensive than institutional care were sincere but based upon mistaken cost estimates. Thus, for many patients, early release from hospitals has not led to successful outcomes.

Despite the faltering of the community psychiatry movement, there has been continued political pressure to provide mental patients with the least restrictive alternative treatment. Institutionalization is seen as a last resort. There is pressure to release mental patients from hospitals as soon as possible and pressure not to hospitalize them at all. The evolution of the mental hospital in the Health Systems period, therefore, has been toward the use of hospitals for shorter periods. However, Greenblatt reports that the rate of first admissions and readmissions per unit of population has slightly increased from the mid-1950s to the late-1960s and early 1970s (36). Nevertheless, mental hospitals continue to be threatened with reduction of funds, lack of community support and possible closure or reduction in size.

For those mental patients who remain in hospital settings, the use of drugs has sometimes led to over-medication or the use of medication without adequate supplemental therapy. Periodic journalistic accounts or occasional lawsuits have revealed that, in some institutions, drugs are used for custodial control rather than as therapeutic instruments.

Treatment Goals. Treatment goals in the Health Systems

period are affected by several factors. First, the uncertain outcomes of drug and other forms of therapy make the formulation of treatment goals difficult. Second, the availability of treatment resources is restricted by political pressures to find cheaper but not necessarily better forms of therapy. Third, patient consent has become a significant force in the establishment of treatment goals. Patient cooperation is a therapeutic asset, but patient consent is a legal and ethical requirement for treatment. Considerable uncertainty exists about how informed consent can be integrated into the formation of treatment goals. This will be discussed further in the section on patient status.

Professional Stance

Authority to Act. One result of the public policy changes sketched above is that the psychiatrist's authority to act has been challenged. The challenges come from several different sources. First, governmental regulation has increasingly moved into clinical as well as economic aspects of practice, requiring professional accountability to peer review as well as regulating payment for services and funding for research. Second, the legal and ethical doctrine of informed consent, long a prominent topic in medical care generally, has been explicitly applied to psychiatry. Redlich and Mollica write that:

> We believe that informed consent is the basis of all psychiatric intervention and without it, no psychiatric intervention can be morally justified. The only exception would be a patient judged incompetent to give his informed consent, preferably by a court. In this situation the state could decide to give informed consent for the patient through proper judicial channels (37).

Maisel, Roth and Lidz (38) trace the legal doctrine of informed consent and reach a similar conclusion. To the extent that informed consent is a basis for psychiatric treatment, the authority of the psychiatrist to act on the basis of scientific knowledge and professional dominance, as in the Therapeutic period, has been diminished.

Third, interprofessional tensions between psychiatrists and other mental health professionals such as psychologists, clinical social workers, marriage and family counselors, and psychiatric nurses, have further eroded the professional dominance of psychiatrists. The current controversy about who is or should be authorized to provide psychotherapy is one manifestation of these tensions.

Fourth, psychiatry has also been under attack from within medicine. Whereas nonmedical critics of psychiatry contend that it has become too technical and scientific, critics from within medicine claim that psychiatry is too "soft" and unscientific. The movement within psychiatry to reestablish credibility within traditional clinical medicine as well as research-oriented scientific medicine is in part a reaction to the multidirectional challenges to the authority of psychiatry.

Professional Rights. Psychiatrists' right to treat has been sharply restricted. Their power to prescribe appropriate treatments has begun to give way to the notion that psychiatrists must negotiate with their patients in an atmosphere of mutuality. Redlich and Mollica claim that "all medical and psychiatric relationships are bound by an obligation to establish a patient-physician or subject-experimenter 'partnership.' This partnership, or working alliance, rather than blind trust or a business-like contract, is offered to the patient as a working solution" (39).

The situation is, in my opinion, still rather unsettled. The metaphors endorsed by Redlich and Mollica are appropriate for some types of relationships but not others. The number of possible relationships that exist defy characterization by a single metaphor such as partnership or the somewhat different notion of working alliance. No single metaphor is rich enough to capture the diverse needs of patients nor the range of services available in psychiatric treatment. Thus the need for negotiation in an atmosphere of mutual respect shaped by governmental regulation puts the rights of psychiatrists to treat or do research in a new and more complex perspective (40).

Professional Responsibilities. As professional rights have become more restricted, professional responsibilities have become more circumscribed. Psychiatrists are less able to prescribe treatments based solely on their determination of the medical needs of patients. Instead, treatment alternatives, if any, must be identified and the psychiatrist must make recommendations. The right to decide treatment has been transferred from the psychiatrist back to the patient. Of course, this conceptual change may not always be exemplified in practice; contrary to the usual rule that theory follows practice, it may be that theory will have a significant influence on future practice. Similarly, the responsibility of psychiatrists to study mental illness scientifically has been subordinated to their responsibility to follow government regulations as well as patient preferences concerning participation in research or experimentation. An additional responsibility imposed upon psychiatrists as a result of increasing judicial scrutiny is the post-*Tarasoff* attitude that psychiatrists have a responsibility to protect society. This movement, though away from patients' rights, is a further limitation on professional discretion. As professional discretion has been restricted, explicit professional responsibilities have expanded.

Patient Status

Competence. In the Custodial period, the mentally ill were presumed incompetent until they proved their competence. In the Therapeutic period, the assumption was that persons with mental illness could be restored to competence. In the Health Systems period, there has been a decided shift toward a presumption of competence until proven incompetent. Several factors have contributed to this change.

Szasz's claim that mental illness is a myth has raised the question of whether there is a tendency to label persons too quickly as mentally ill and incompetent. Even if one is not a Szaszian, it is possible to acknowledge that the tendency to equate mental illness with nonresponsibility may be a mistake. Mental illness, even defined more broadly than Szasz would permit, does not necessarily imply incompetence.

Another factor that helps to account for the shift in patient status is the impact of the informed consent doctrine and the underlying ethical orientation toward personal autonomy. Persons are presumed competent even if they are mentally ill, unless their conduct shows that they are incompetent. For example, persons suffering from mental illness can be viewed as competent to consent to treatment if they display a minimum degree of understanding of their needs (41). As long as a person's choices appear to be consistent with his/her apparent needs, including need for mental health treatment, competence is not likely to be seriously questioned.

Still another trend contributing to the presumption of competence is that the standard for involuntary civil commitment has shifted from psychiatric discretion to patient behavior. In many states, involuntary civil commitment requires evidence that persons suffering from a mental disorder *act* in ways that are dangerous to themselves or others. The shift has been from a judgment about the persons's mental *state* to an assessment of *behavior*.

Needs. Unlike the Custodial period, when the mentally ill were segregated from the rest of society, the Health Systems period emphasizes integration of the mentally ill into society. As a result of the use of psychopharmacologics and the declining number of mental hospitals, persons with mental illness are encouraged to seek reentry into functional roles in society. Although resources for rehabilitation of the mentally ill have been inadequate, the desirability of this goal is widely endorsed. It is felt that the mentally ill need reintegration even if they function with handicaps. Just as the physically and developmentally disabled have sought to overcome legal and social obstacles to their exercise of basic rights, the mentally ill have begun to seek similar support. At present, the mentally ill are much less effective in exerting political influence because they are not well-organized, but their need for tolerance and acceptance is as great as those who have other disabilities.

Rights. Consistent with the increased emphasis on the right of the mentally ill to give informed consent to psychiatric care is the increasing interest in their right to select from among alternative available treatments or even to refuse treatment. In response to charges that some psychiatrists have imposed unwanted and dangerous treatments on unwilling patients, a few courts have recognized the right of involuntary but competent patients as well as voluntary patients to refuse treatment (42). Persons who are mentally ill and not dangerous to others are considered to be competent enough to refuse psychiatric care, especially if the treatment proposed has undesirable side effects. The recognition of this right brings out the difficulties with a system of involuntary civil commitment that confuses the protection of society with the need for psychiatric care. A person who needs psychiatric care may nevertheless have a right to refuse treatment. This shift is further evidence of the decline of psychiatric discretion and the rise of patient autonomy.

Responsibilities. In keeping with the increased emphasis on patient competence, we are beginning to see attention directed to patient responsibilities. These include the responsibility to co-operate in treatment and, in some instances, to participate with the treatment personnel in developing a treatment plan. This can occur in hospital settings, behavior modification or individual psychotherapy. Patients are playing a more active role in their own psychiatric care just as they have in other forms of health care. This trend is by no means a radical transformation, but there are signs that change is taking place. Further evidence for the trend towards increased recognition of patients' responsibilities lies in the fact that persons who are mentally ill are no longer automatically excused from responsibility for immoral or illegal conduct.

FUTURE DIRECTIONS

As the Health Systems period matures, we have begun to see more concrete and often conflictual interactions among health, legal and political systems, not only in America but also throughout the world. It is difficult to predict the shape and direction of future change, but it does seem inevitable that the general trend toward legal regulation and political control of health systems will be felt quite strongly in psychiatry. For this reason, it is especially urgent that persons interested in psychiatry devote increasing attention to ethical issues. The substantive and often perplexing problems involved in examining and revising fundamental assumptions and values must be confronted directly and thoughtfully by psychiatrists, other health professionals, and their critics. These explorations must not be conducted in isolation. Rather, they require an atmosphere of common concern about issues and mutual respect for different assumptions, methods and values. In this way, it may be possible to prevent psychiatry from being buffeted about by the gusts of political winds and to prevent it from being hopelessly buried in legal procedures and bureaucracy.

REFERENCES

1. Wittgensein, L.: *Philosophical Investigations,* Section 127. New York: Macmillan & Co., 1953, p. 50.
2. See Waismann, F.: How I See Philosophy, reprinted in *Logical Positivism* (A. J. Ayer, ed.). Glencoe, IL: The Free Press, 1959, pp. 345-380.
3. My primary sources for the historical material are Albert Deutsch's classic, *The Mentally Ill in America,* and Milton Greenblatt's comprehensive historical-conceptual synthesis, The Evolution of Models of Mental Health Care and Treatment, Chapter 7 of *Psychopolitics.* The division of American psychiatry into three historical periods is modified from Fritz Redlich's unpublished paper, The Past in Perspective, an address given at the 25th Anniversary of the Foundations Fund for Research in Psychiatry. I have also profited a great deal from conversations with Doctors Greenblatt and Redlich.
4. Magaro, P. A., Gripp, R. and McDowell, D. J.: *The Mental Health Industry, A Cultural Phenomenon.* New York: John Wiley & Sons, 1978, p. 27.
5. As quoted by Albert Deutsch, *op. cit.,* p. 207.
6. Deutsch, *ibid.,* p. 217.
7. Greenblatt, M.: *Psychopolitics.* New York: Grune and Stratton, 1978, p. 100.
8. See Foucault, M.: *Madness and Civilization.* New York: Vintage Books, 1973.
9. McIntyre, A.: *A Short History of Ethics.* New York: Macmillan, 1960, p. 247.
10. See Winslade, W. J.: The Juvenile Courts: From Idealism to Hypocrisy, *Social Theory and Practice,* Fall, 1974, pp. 181-199.
11. *Report of the President's Commission on Mental Health,* Washington, D.C.: U.S. Government Printing Office, 1978.
12. Redlich, *op cit.,* p. 2.

64   *Law and Ethics in the Practice of Psychiatry*

13. Greenblatt, *op. cit.*, p. 102.
14. *Ibid.*, p. 100.
15. The Mental Health Industry, *op. cit.*, p. 36.
16. Redlich, *op. cit.*, p. 1.
17. Greenblatt, *op. cit.*, p. 101.
18. The well-known case of Kenneth Donaldson, though occurring after the Custodial period, illustrates the potential abuse of authority by both hospital superintendents (in the *Donaldson* case, a pediatrician rather than a pyschiatrist) and a treating psychiatrist. Not only did the physicians have authority to decide, this authority, though technically subject to review, was in fact unchallenged for many years. (*Donaldson v. O'Connor*, U.S. Supreme Court, No. 74-8, June 26, 1975.)
19. Greenblatt, p. 101.
20. Particularly electro-convulsive therapy, insulin hypoglycemia and lobotomy.
21. This recalls a similar mood in the nineteenth century.
22. Greenblatt, p. 103.
23. *Ibid.*, p. 103.
24. Redlich, pp. 4, 5.
25. Greenblatt, p. 103.
26. See Frank, J.: *Law and the Modern Mind;* and Arnold, T.: *The Folk Lore of Capitalism.*
27. Freud, A.: Barriers to Rational Decision Making. In *Experimentation with Human Beings* (J. Katz, ed.), N.Y., 1972, pp. 635-637.
28. Redlich, p. 4.
29. *Ibid.*, p. 5.
30. *Ibid.*, p. 6.
31. Recently, a bill has been introduced in the California legislature (AB 3382) to create a licensure for doctors of mental health. The law would specifically authorize such persons to prescribe certain kinds of drugs even though the mental health doctors are not M.D.'s.
32. Redlich, F. and Mollica, R. F.: Overview: Ethical Issues in Contemporary Psychiatry, *The American Journal of Psychiatry*, Vol. 133, #2, February 1976.
33. See Winslade, W. J.: Critical Study of Paul Ramsey's *The Patient as a Person, Institute of Human Values in Medicine, Report of Fellows,* 1974.
34. *The Hastings Center Report,* Vol. 9, #4, August, 1979, p. 17.
35. Drugs for the Mind: Psychiatry's Newest Weapon, *Newsweek,* November 12, 1979, p. 98 *et seq.*
36. Greenblatt, p. 163.
37. Redlich and Mollica, p. 125.
38. Toward a Model of the Legal Doctrine of Informed Consent, *American Journal of Psychiatry*, Vol. 134, March, 1977, pp. 285-289.
39. Redlich and Mollica, p. 125.
40. See Winslade, W. J.: Patient and Physician: Who Is Responsible for What? *Contemporary Surgery*, Nov., 1978, p. 39 ff.
41. Roth, L.: A Commitment Law for Patients, Doctors and Lawyers, *The*

American Journal of Psychiatry, Vol. 136, #9, September, 1979, pp. 1121-1127.
42. *Rogers, et al. v. Okin et al.,* USDA — Mass., C. A. #75-1610T, Oct 29, 1979. Both *Rogers* in Massachusetts and the *Rennie* case in New Jersey (1979) held that patients may not be given psychotropic drugs without their consent except in emergencies.

Part II

CLINICAL ISSUES

3

Privacy and Confidentiality

Jerome S. Beigler, M.D.

INTRODUCTION

This essay will consider the privacy and confidentiality problems in the psychiatrist-patient relationship which result from the following factors: 1) the increasing proportion of treatment paid for by third-party carriers such as health insurance firms and government agencies; 2) the psychiatrist's need to protect him/herself against malpractice litigation; 3) the trend towards using psychiatrists as agents of social control; and 4) the pressure by patients for access to their records. Coping with these realities requires an organized set of strategies and tactics in regard to record-keeping, responses to third-party requirements, and recent judicial and legislative developments.

Let us consider first the complications brought by the health insurance industry.

HEALTH INSURANCE

A phenomenon of our time has been the burgeoning of health insurance coverage. There have been problems with cost control even in the nonpsychiatric medical disciplines, where diagnoses, test procedures and durations of illnesses are relatively finite and statistically predictable. Psychiatric illness presents actuarial and fiduciary problems that are only beginning to be defined and answered. Not only is a psychiatric illness relatively intangible, but it can also be treated by several alternative approaches and often has an indeterminate prognosis. In addition, a psychiatric diagnosis still carries a stigma. A further complication is that a few patients and practitioners have taken unethical advantage of these imprecise parameters to their profit. The insurance industry, on the other hand, has sometimes responded harshly and exploited the situation in its own resourceful ways. Moreover, large segments of the public put psychiatric coverage low on their list of insurance priorities, so that coverage tends to be limited to a self-selected population of individuals who feel they may need psychiatric care.

One of the early privacy problems that surfaced as a result of insurance benefits utilization was breach of confidentiality. Health information was often leaked through the personnel offices of the employer. Not only was there a loss of privacy, but sometimes a patient would learn for the first time of a malignancy or schizophrenia from the gratuitous solicitude of a well-meaning friend at work (1) or from receiving a copy of the payment report from the carrier to the employer.

Another complication of using insurance benefits was that a person's employment and career might be affected by his/her record as a psychiatric patient. In order not to jeopardize their immediate employment or future careers, civil service employers, military personnel, corporate executives, politicians, and teachers soon learned not to use their insurance coverage for psychiatric treatment (2, 3, 4, 5). Because of a sophisticated awareness of the potential benefits to the individual, the employer and society, a few private corporations, government agencies, and boards of education actually encourage needed psychiatric treatment, but most employers view the development of a psychiatric problem as an unfortunate complication in the assessment of an employee, especially for promotion.

A simple way to minimize the problem of unauthorized disclosures is to by-pass the employer's personnel office by routing insurance claims directly to the office of the carrier's medical director, where geographic distance and training of personnel will tend to protect confidentiality. Several large corporations have implemented such a program successfully: The employer receives only periodic statistical analyses of insurance usage, and individual patients remain anonymous (6).

Another insurance-related problem results from difficulties in cost-accountability. In an effort to control costs, psychiatric benefits have often been severely curtailed or eliminated (7). Psychiatric insurance benefits are monitored closely, and a large amount of seemingly unnecessary information is required for claims processing. Requests are made for submission of entire hospital charts; state auditors invade hospital record rooms and private-office files; detailed claim-questionnaires have become common. Is all this necessary? The demands for information are motivated by a quest for effective answers in a complex, bewildering field with many internal contradictions. One of an insurance executive's major responsibilities is to predict benefit utilization so that optimal rates can be set. Psychiatry presents an actuarial dilemma. Carriers must be able to predict levels of cash reserves in order to set premium rates and to meet competition. Psychiatry seemingly provides only a quagmire, but the stakes are large and potential profits could be significant if one could only find a formula.

In a new field, an enterprising executive must experiment. The results are not always pleasant. In the recent past, a promising young insurance officer with family experience in psychiatry, motivated to succeed and also to provide coverage for an under-insured segment of the population, convinced his superiors to introduce a psychiatric-benefit package oriented to an upper middle-class clientele, who would probably have the sophistication and time to be interested (8). True to his assessment, the policy sold well. Prospects seemed bright—until the claims began to arrive. In two years, the programs lost several million dollars. There were a few cases of apparent abuse, but the real miscalculation was an actuarial one. Lack of experience had prevented an accurate assessment of the latent need. Also, the more sophisticated and successful families shrewdly selected the benefit program, being aware of their latent need and potential benefit, a procedure which resulted in a fiduciary debacle. The policy was taken off the market, and the unfortunate executive found work with a smaller firm.

Of interest were the defensive maneuvers made by the stricken carrier in an understandable effort to cut losses. Processing of claims was delayed resourcefully; additional information was repetitively requested; claims were indiscriminately denied; new questionnaires requesting intimate and irrelevant information were devised (which included clinically meaningless questions about the transference). Experience was gained in negotiating some of the efforts made by the carrier to revoke its contract. Personal phone calls protesting the amount of information newly required sometimes were effective; persistence sometimes worked, but in a large number of cases only expensive litigation prevailed. This is an extreme example, but the experience is instructive.

On the one hand, carriers have a legitimate need for adequate information to process claims effectively; on the other hand, psychiatric patients, in order to benefit optimally from treatment, particularly psychotherapy and psychoanalysis, must disclose to their psychiatrists sensitive information, which could be injurious to privacy and career, if revealed to others. The dilemma is where to draw the line between two countervailing rights. Complicating the problem are the human failings of patient, physician and carrier. Insurance companies would like to have complete access to all information and assure patient confidentiality. Physicians and patients would prefer to maintain doctor-patient confidentiality, knowing that despite the best of carrier intentions, information once recorded in insurance files becomes vulnerable to discovery. Unfortunately once such records become accessible, innumerable problems may develop, such as unreasonable denial of claims, peremptory cancellation of insurance, loss of employment, impairment of career and invasion of privacy (1-4).

Another specific example will help illustrate some of the problems. Blue Cross-Blue Shield of Washington, D.C. devised a

Mental and Nervous Disease Utilization Cost Study (MAN-DUCS). They developed special claim forms in an effort to research cost-accountability in its coverage of the Federal Employees Health Benefit Plan (FEP). The forms included questions regarding alcoholism, drugs, depression and suicide. Assurances were given about confidentiality. Vigorous protests by patients and psychiatrists ensued (9-11). Patients feared leakage of sensitive information to employers and loss of privacy. Blue Cross-Blue Shield inadvertently did disclose information on some patients, while keeping "V.I.P." files under even greater "security" than ordinary files. Also, the research results did not disclose criteria for accurate monitoring of utilization. As the result of continued negotiations and the threat of a class-action suit, the MANDUCS forms were withdrawn and a simple claims form requiring only innocuous information was substituted (1-11). Ninety percent of FEP claims are now processed with the new form. The remainder require more detailed information according to local carrier criteria, including local peer review.

From this example, one learned that even a large insurance company was amenable to education, persuasion, and negotiation. Also, fears that unless detailed information was given, insurance benefits would be stopped proved groundless (10). It is understandable that carriers are under pressure to monitor utilization of the mental health care benefits effectively. The situation is new, and the stakes are high. The Blues' FEP insures 600,000 federal workers and dependents in the Washington area and 5.9 million nationwide. The Blues paid $108 million in mental health payments in 1976 (10). Insurance executives have to learn the professional intricacies of a complex new area. More than others, psychiatric patients bring with them complications regarding constitutional rights to privacy, civil liberties, social stigma and employability. Intelligent insurance executives have responded as creatively as possible, but it is the responsibility of psychiatrists to bring information and effective persuasion to the educational process. Confidentiality is a new problem superimposed on an already difficult administrative challenge. In my view, cost-effective insurance for psychiatric problems and confidentiality in the interest of patients can be compatible.

Let us now turn to a third example of a confidentiality problem with insurance, namely the CHAMPUS (Civilian Health and Medical Program of the Uniformed Services) program. It covers dependents of uniformed personnel, retired personnel and their dependents, as well as the surviving dependents of deceased personnel. Administered as a direct component of the secretariat of the Secretary of Defense according to specific federal laws and regulations, it is subject to direct congressional funding and oversight. Between six-and-a-half and seven million dependents and retirees are covered. In fiscal year 1977, the CHAMPUS budget was about $586 million, of which $88 million (15%) was for mental health services (12).

CHAMPUS provided the most complete psychiatric coverage of any plan, but was the victim of unconscionable exploitation by resourceful providers, especially in facilities for the residential treatment of children and adolescents, thereby triggering congressional investigations and cutbacks (1974). As a result, CHAMPUS and the APA contracted for a peer-review program aimed at providing benefits on a cost-effective basis (12). A Mental Health Treatment Report (MHTR) form was designed to implement the program. Again, more sensitive information was required than seemed necessary for claims processing. Complete dossiers on some patients would eventually be accumulated in the files of fiscal intermediaries and in the office of CHAMPUS. The disinclination of the uniformed services to maintain psychiatric confidentiality is notorious (13, 14). Federal regulations mandate dissemination of CHAMPUS patient records without consent in some situations (15). Negotiations between CHAMPUS and various components of the APA resulted in modification of some of the objectionable features in the insurance plans (16, 17). Acceptable protection of privacy applicable to CHAMPUS alcohol and drug-abuse patients (18), however, could not be applied to other CHAMPUS patients for bureaucratic and technical reasons.

Although two federal programs—Alcohol and Drug Abuse (18),

Medicare and Medicaid Fraud Abuse Control (19)—protect the confidentiality of patient records, the APA-CHAMPUS peer-review protocol allows for the accumulation of sensitive clinical material in the files of fiscal intermediaries and in the office of CHAMPUS. Such material is usually sent only to peer-reviewers, who are trained to maintain confidentiality, whereas the CHAMPUS program mandates the routine use of peer-review material through claims-processing (fiscal) channels. This is a considerable regressive step, compared even to the MANDUCS program, and it constitutes an enhancement of an already-accelerating erosion of confidentiality and the doctor-patient relationship.

These problems could be avoided if the CHAMPUS protocol were changed to process peer-review material only through peer-review channels. A prototype arrangement is already in operation between CHAMPUS and the National Capitol Medical Foundation (a PSRO) in Washington, D.C. (20, 21).

Shortly after the CHAMPUS Peer Review Project was adopted (22), a similar program was instituted with Aetna Life and Casualty Insurance Company, using the same MHTR forms processed through the office of Aetna's medical director. When peer review seems warranted, the record will be sanitized, sent to the APA Peer Review Project office for coding and distribution to three members of the group for review. Their reports will be collated by the APA, reviewer-identifiers removed, and only the review-recommendations sent to Aetna for disposition (23).

Because the Aetna project involves only the private sector, there are no federal regulations to restrict claims-processing and peer-review. Only the laws of the local jurisdictions apply. Because of patient concerns over having so much sensitive information on file, and therefore discoverable, the Washington (DC) Psychiatric Society took the initiative in protesting potential breaches of confidentiality and a centralized peer-review system (24). It was pointed out that the 1978 District of Columbia Mental Health Information Act prohibits the disclosure of detailed mental health patient information to insurance companies, so that filling out an MHTR by a District of Columbia psychiatrist could be illegal and actionable (25). A similar restriction on such disclosures is provided by Virginia law (26).

As of December, 1979, 6700 MHTRs had been received by Aetna's medical director, but only 175 were selected for peer review. Thus, only 2.6% of cases were considered suspicious of over-utilization, illustrating that the sensitive information in MHTRs was used primarily for claims-processing. Because of the administrative burden imposed by the accumulation of so much paper, the insurer hopes to devise simpler criteria for identifying suspicious cases (27).

A potential solution to the confidentiality problems in insurance-claim processing is to establish an independent local peer-review program as is already in operation in Washington, D.C. for CHAMPUS inpatients (21) and in use in the Denver district-branch peer-review committee for Blue Cross-Blue Shield outpatients (28).

Four insurance-related problems regarding confidentiality have been considered. Various strategies and tactics to cope with these problems have been illustrated by the narration of actual experiences. The individual practitioner should acquaint him/herself with local confidentiality and privilege laws, consult with colleagues and legal counsel, appropriately discuss these matters with patients, and support his/her own district branch, the APA and the AMA so that they can influence legislation and litigation. On the strategic level, it is important to have effective laws enacted (29), as illustrated by their potency in the APA-Aetna problem, and by their absence in the APA-CHAMPUS project. Such laws are enacted as the result of intervention by district branches, usually in cooperation with state medical societies. Federal legislation requires APA interventions. The first prerequisite, then, is to have a legislative umbrella to provide legal protection. The next is to support one's district branch's intervention in appropriate litigation. District-branch efforts at establishing peer-review arrangements with local insurers should also be encouraged. Effective peer review can raise professional standards of both provider and insurer. Thus, the second level of protection of confidentiality is to have an effective peer-review structure. On an individual basis, it is sometimes effective, when an insurance claim form requires excessive information, to call the insurance company's claims manager for clarification and explanation. Even if there is no immediately apparent result, the inquiry together with those of many others may help insurance personnel better to understand psychiatric treatment. There have been many cases in which simply not answering controversial questions, or even replying that an answer would violate the privacy rights of the patient have not interfered with payment.

In the actual filling out of a claim form requiring extensive responses, it is wise to have the complete participation of the patient, who should know what information is being forwarded to the insurer. In less complicated cases, the completed form should be sent to the patient for review before it is sent on.

When the insurer insists on disclosure of information not relevant to actual claims processing, some patients may be willing to initiate litigation to prevent unreasonable disclosures. In a few cases, as in the MANDUCS situation, a class action suit may be feasible. Specific actions will depend on the legislative, judicial and legal ambience of the local jurisdiction, as illustrated by the situations in the District of Columbia and Virginia.

THE KEEPING OF RECORDS

The problems involved in record-keeping may best be introduced by a personal clinical anecdote. Several years ago, in responding to an insurance claim questionnaire, I outlined the development of my patient's character from his childhood on. The carrier denied the patient's claim on the basis that his condition had been present from childhood, and preexisting conditions were not covered. I no longer write more than is minimally required on insurance forms or on patient records.

In another instance, a progress note on one of my patients stated that the patient was improving and it was appropriate to initiate discharge planning. Later, the insurance company refused payment as of the date of the progress note on the basis that subsequent hospitalization was only for custodial care pending the arrangement of finding a companion. Hospital personnel have now learned not to make such entries.

Experiences such as these are common throughout the country and illustrate how clinical recordings, teaching and potential research have been adventitiously changed in response to the economics of third-party payments.

Another problem regarding the keeping of records has to do with patients' access to their records. Concern with access to records resulted, in part, from the surfacing of errors in computerized data banks regarding financial credit. Also, school and medical records containing information about childhood illnesses or family background proved in some cases to have deleterious effects on careers (30). Initial legislative responses included the Buckley amendment of 1975 (31), in which Congress authorized access to school records by student or parent. The Privacy Act of 1974 established the Privacy Protection Study Commission which worked effectively for two years, uncovering intolerable credit agency practices, the unauthorized sharing of health and insurance information between carriers such as through the Medical Information Bureau, and the illicit insurance information industry supported by the insurance carriers which was exposed by Denver District Attorney Dale Tooley (30). A similar scandal regarding the illicit trading of medical information involving the Royal Canadian Mounted Police was uncovered in Canada (6, 32). The public has become progressively more concerned with the inappropriate use of personal records in our increasingly information-hungry computerized society. Together with the patients' rights movement, there has resulted a democratic demand that citizens participate in the shaping of their own destinies. This includes knowing what is in one's medical record.

Clinicians know that medical records traditionally have not been available to patients. There is some objective validity to this practice, in that clinical information can be misinterpreted by laity. Some information, such as diagnoses of malignancy or schizophrenia could be injurious if prematurely or tactlessly disclosed, and some information in the record may have been given in confidence by third parties to help the patient's management. Thus, a problem is again posed by two countervailing rights; the right of a patient to see his record and the right of a physician to protect his patient and third parties.

In the Buckley amendment, provision is made that a student or parent may have access to the school record, but if the medical record contains information of potential harm to the student, it is referred to a professional of the student's choice for screening and interpretation (31).

The APA Model Law on Confidentiality also has a section on patient access to clinical records (33). It was felt that access to records by a patient in a working therapeutic relationship could be used constructively to foster the treatment. However, in those instances in which information might be injurious, the patient may appoint another clinician as a "clinical mediator" who will then review, interpret, or refuse to disclose the record to the patient. Should the mediator refuse disclosure and the patient persist in requesting access, he may seek judicial relief. The judge, after *in camera* review of the record, will then determine whether to disclose or not (33). A similar set of provisos was enacted in the 1978 District of Columbia Mental Health Information Act (34). Other states also have passed statutes allowing patient access to clinical records. Most access statutes also provide for the correction of misinformation in the record, or for inclusion of a statement from the patient that there is a difference of opinion about the validity of the information.

There is one further set of strategies to protect a psychiatrist's records from counterproductive access by patients or third parties (insurers, courts, adversaries). At the 1974 Key Biscayne Conference on Confidentiality, the American Medical Records Association recommended the establishment of two sets of records on each patient—one the official record containing factual data and notes on the patient, the other the "personal notes of the therapist which would contain research data, information from third parties given in confidence and clinical conjectures." Access would be provided to the official record, but not to the personal notes (35). The background for this recommendation comes from legal practice. Lawyers are provided with legal protection of their "work product" in that an adversary is not allowed to subpoena a lawyer's notes containing the results of legal research, strategy planning and information from his/her client.

This seems a feasible idea and was incorporated into the APA Model Law (36) with provisos that personal notes are not discoverable. This has already been enacted in Illinois (37) and Washington, D.C. (38). In Illinois, personal notes are not discoverable; in Washington, personal notes are not part of a client's record, access is "strictly and absolutely limited" to the professional and shall not be disclosed except to the degree needed in malpractice litigation (38). The Illinois law apparently provides absolute privilege to personal notes; the Washington law provides an exception. "Personal notes" is an innovative concept, the practicality of which will have to be tested with experience. Although it may be cumbersome at first, it seems to work well. Thus far there have been two important Illinois court tests in which the personal notes of an examining psychiatrist were judged to be nondiscoverable (39).

One should also be reminded that it is both ethically and legally incumbent on the psychiatrist to maintain confidentiality of a patient's communications to him. The APA Code of Ethics stresses this obligation (40) and even in jurisdictions without specific privilege or confidentiality laws, common law or public policy dictates the legal obligation to maintain confidentiality (41). There is case law to the effect that a physician who makes unauthorized disclosures to a patient's employer is liable for resulting damages for invasion of privacy (42, 43). Also, a physician's unauthorized submission of a report on his patient to a doctor employed by the patient's adversary in litigation was judged a breach of confidentiality (44). Similarly, a physician furnishing information to an insurance company without the insured patient's authorization was found to be in violation of confidence (45). Federal rules and regulations regarding unauthorized disclosures of alcohol and drug-abuse patient records are particularly strict and include specific penalties (18).

Legal criteria for publication of clinical data has recently been defined in the important New York case of *Doe v. Roe* in which Judge Stecher defined legal parameters of informed consent, adequate disguise and scientific value as the criteria governing such disclosures (41).

In most jurisdictions, if deemed in the patient's interest, a subpoena usually can be successfully contested. Recently Dr. Loren Roth successfully resisted a subpoena for disclosure of a mother's psychiatric hospitalization records in a child custody case on the basis of a state constitutional right to privacy even though the records were not deemed protected by a privilege statute (46). As can be seen, the question of privilege of communications is highly technical and has been discussed in more detail in a recent study (47).

Another question concerns the disposition of a deceased psychiatrist's records. In a New York case, it was found that although medical records are the property of the physician, the destruction of his records as provided in his will was considered against public policy and invalid; the executor was to make the records available to the succeeding physicians of the patients involved (42, 48). In another case, however, it was determined the original records belonged to the estate and only copies could be sent to physicians authorized by the patients (49).

It is recommended that the executor of a deceased psychiatrist's estate arrange to notify the patients of the psychiatrist's death and that records are available for transfer to an authorized physician. After six months, the unclaimed records should be stored in a repository for a period of five years before being destroyed. There is a responsibility to keep the records available in case of future litigation by the patients or their estates such as in future personal injury suits or contested wills. The case law on this subject is minimal, as is statutory direction. More precise resolution of the problem will have to await further jurisprudential clarification.

RECENT LEGISLATIVE AND JUDICIAL ACTIONS

As discussed in detail in another study (47), there have been several developments in the past few years that complicate the ability of a psychiatrist to maintain the confidentiality of his patient's communications. There seems to be a trend towards using psychiatrists and psychiatric records for purposes of social control. It is reasonable to expect physicians to report communicable diseases and gunshot wounds. More debatable is the problem of using psychiatric records in the assessment of driver's license applications, drug abusers, gun permit applicants and child abusers. Federal rules and regulations have been designed to protect patient privacy in alcohol and drug-abuse treatment programs (18), but there have been several instances in which police and auditors have ignored federal regulations, forced access to records and undermined the clinical effectiveness of the programs (47, 50, 51). Litigation and formal inquires have been used to counter such peremptory police incursions (47, 51).

More complex and subtle is the 1976 California *Tarasoff* case (47, 52, 53). Due to the idiosyncracies of California evidence law, the state Supreme Court found that in some circumstances, a psychiatrist has an obligation to inform intended victims of a patient's possible aggression. Technically such a potential duty to warn a victim applies only in California, but many of our colleagues, lawyers and judges over the country have interpreted the decision to mandate a duty to warn in other jurisdictions as well. In a recent Illinois case, an appellate court judge found there is no duty to warn in Illinois (54), but a New Jersey judge accepted the validity of *Tarasoff* and ordered a similar New Jersey case to trial (55).

The APA Committee on Confidentiality finds that *Tarasoff* imposes a dilemma remediable only by corrective legislation (56). A proposed position statement points out that there is no unequivocal mandate to warn a potential victim; that maintaining the clinical therapeutic relationship is potentially the most effective method of defusing a patient's loss of control over his aggressions; and that a psychiatrist is not expected to make infallible predictions of dangerousness. However, there must be documentation that one was not negligent; consultation with colleagues and/or lawyers can be useful in this regard. Only if the patient does not respond to treatment or will not accept hospitalization is it necessary to solicit help from family, friends or the police. Only if all these measures are ineffective would it be necessary to consider warning a potential victim; however, even warning a victim does not end the problem, because the victim usually cannot change his/her circumstances, or may become violent against the patient, or may initiate action against the psychiatrist in case the warning proved unnecessary and caused the supposed victim distress or illness. In addition, the patient may have a cause of action for breach of confidentiality. Furthermore, in California as in other parts of the country, it is difficult because of legal restrictions to hospitalize a patient involuntarily should he require it. Thus, the APA Committee on Confidentiality sees the *Tarasoff* decision as presenting an impossible clinical and legal dilemma. The committee recommends vigorous efforts at remedial legislation and, in the meantime, suggests that psychiatrists carefully document all their evaluations and consult with other professionals when necessary (56). In Illinois and in the APA Model Law on Confidentiality, provision is made so that potential victims of a patient's aggression may be warned at the clinician's discretion (33, 37). As a result of *Tarasoff*, a recent survey has demonstrated that there has been a significant erosion in the psychiatrist-patient relationship (57). Psychiatrists report patients do not now enter treatment when they may have to reveal their aggressive fantasies, lest their therapist disclose their confidences. Similarly some patients have left treatment rather than reveal their impulses, and other patients stay in treatment but do not disclose aggressive material (58). *Tarasoff* and its consequences illustrate the progressive erosion of a clinician's capacity to assure confidentiality, thereby impairing his ability to be optimally helpful. The case also illustrates the need to document clinical and legal considerations that lead to specific decisions in the treatment of a patient with aggressive impulses.

Further evidence of the general erosion of psychiatry's ability to help its patients is provided by the U.S. Supreme Court's May 31, 1978 decision in the case of *Zurcher v. Stanford Daily News* (59). The court upheld the validity of Zurcher, Palo Alto's chief of police, having obtained a warrant in 1971 to search the premises of the Stanford University student newspaper for pictures of a student attack on the police. A warrant is usually issued against those suspected of a crime. Judicial sanction for the search of innocent third parties is new. *Zurcher* applies not only to newspaper offices, but to any office or home. *Zurcher* would have enabled Nixon's "plumbers" to officially search Dr. Fielding's offices for Ellsberg's records rather than having to burglarize (60). Zurcher, shortly after his search of the newspaper, also searched the office and home of a Palo Alto psychiatrist for the records of a patient who had complained to the police of a sexual assault. Not only were the doctor's records searched, but so were those of her husband, who is a well-known scientist (60, 61). Moreover, warrants were recently executed to search the offices of the Santa Clara County's public defender (61) and also a methadone clinic in San Francisco (51), even though the latter is supposedly protected by federal rules and regulations (18). Similarly, in 1978, Hawaii passed Act 105 allowing warrants for the search of providers' offices when it is "in the public interest" to monitor Medicaid programs (61). The statute has been declared unconstitutional by a federal district court, but the decision may be appealed (62).

A search warrant is a potent law-enforcement device. In contrast to a subpoena, which can be contested, a search warrant, once issued, cannot be resisted. The newspaper industry responded to *Zurcher* vigorously (63) and several bills were introduced to protect their interests (64), but there is little assurance that there will be legislation to protect the premises of the professions or laity. The American Bar Association at its August, 1979 meeting refused to support any protective legislation (65).

To add further to our discomfort is the appearance of a series of bills in Congress heralded as legislation to protect the privacy of citizens as recommended by the Privacy Protection Study Commission (30, 66, 67, 68). Unfortunately, all the new bills under the guise of protecting privacy actually are detailed "discovery" bills. They eliminate whatever local state statutory protection of confidentiality there is, provide for access to physicians' and psychiatrists' records by law enforcement agencies by means not only of subpoenas, search warrants and summonses, but also by a simple "formal request." Patients need not be notified of such access and detailed instructions are provided to the law enforcement agencies on how to access medical records (69, 70). It is an Orwellian development that requires vigorous opposition (69, 70) in concert with other professional organizations. The AMA has recommended that the legislation not be passed and that local state statutes be allowed to prevail (71, 72).

Three more recent developments highlight even further the urgency and extent of this trend. Senator Kennedy introduced S. 1612, the FBI Charter Act of 1979, which contains a "physician-informant" provision purporting to restrict the FBI's use of physicians as informants, but could be used to coerce confidential information, and allows free access to the insurance company records. Secondly, President Carter in his State of the Union Address advocated the removal of restraints on our intelligence agencies (73, 74). Thirdly, the Federal Register of January 2, 1980 contains a notice of intent to introduce fifteen changes in the Confidentiality of Alcohol and Drug Abuse Patient Records regulations (75). The proposed changes are in the direction of eliminating confidentiality. If enacted the whole alcohol and drug abuse program could be vitiated.

The sequence of: 1) deliberate breach of federal regulations protecting alcohol and drug abuse treatment programs, 2) the *Tarasoff* decision, 3) the *Zurcher* decision, 4) Hawaii Act 105, 5) the President's so-called medical-record privacy bills that actually provide unlimited access to medical records by law enforcement agencies, 6) the FBI Charter Act, 7) the President's State of the Union Address advocating loosening of strictures on intelligence agencies and 8) the intended changes in the Confidentiality of Alcohol and Drug Abuse Patient Records regulations, warn us of the progressive erosion of privacy and confidentiality that increasingly will disable the psychiatric profession.

One is reminded of the fact that in Uruguay, a psychiatrist who does not notify the government of the political activities of his/her patients is imprisoned for collusion; similarly the abuses of psychiatry in totalitarian countries is well-known (76). As Alexis de Tocqueville warned: " 'If the private rights of an individual are violated . . . the manners of a nation are corrupted, putting the whole community in jeopardy' " (77).

SUMMARY

In summary, we have examined the privacy and confidentiality problems resulting from the idiosyncratic needs of the insurance industry providing psychiatric benefits. These problems are significant in themselves, but also foreshadow the problems to be expected when national health insurance is enacted. We also reviewed the problems in record-keeping and suggested tactics for protecting patient confidentiality, minimizing the risk of malpractice suits and providing patients with access to their records. Also discussed were recent judicial and legislative developments which form a pattern of progressive erosions of the doctor-patient relationship so that clinical effectiveness is impaired and physicians are used as agents of police control. The latter development is ominous not only for the practice of our profession but is a significant threat to our democratic system of government.

REFERENCES

1. Grossman, M. (chairman): Confidentiality and Third Parties. *A Report of the APA Task Force on Confidentiality as it Relates to Third Parties.* Task Force Report 9. Washington, D.C.: American Psychiatric Association, June, 1975, pp. 53-59.
2. Beigler, J. S.: Statement to supplement testimony given on May 20, 1976 in Washington, D.C. to the Privacy Protection Study Commission concerning privacy problems created by the record-keeping practices of insurers and other institutions of the insurance industry.
3. Hitchings, B. (Ed.): Psychiatric records may be used against you. Personal Business. *Business Week,* August 23, 1976, pp. 73-74.
4. Beigler, J. S.: Psychiatry and confidentiality. *Amer. J. Forensic Psychiatry* 1:7-19, 1978. Also in: *Hearings before the Subcommittee on the Constitution of the Committee on the Judiciary,* United States Senate, Ninety-fifth Congress, Second Session, on S. 3162. A Bill to Secure and Protect the Freedom of Individuals from Unwarranted Intrusions by Persons Acting under Color of Law, Washington, D.C., U.S. Government Printing Office, 1979, pp. 254-61.
5. Report to APA Committee on Confidentiality, August, 1979.
6. Aldrich, R. F. (Ed.): *New Approaches. A Report on the Emerging Revolution in Health Records Policy.* Washington, D.C., National

Commission on Confidentiality of Health Records (NCCHR), June, 1979, pp. 30-37.
7. Herrington, B. S.: Blue Cross, Blue Shield tighten psychiatric coverage in East, West. *Psychiatric News,* September 7, 1979, pp. 1, 6, 17; 1, 7 20-21.
8. Details available on request. Information derived during a negotiating session, 1976.
9. Letter from P. R. Friedman, director of the Mental Health Law Project to R. J. Luehrs, Senior Director of Operations, FEP Program, Blue Cross and Blue Shield, Washington, D.C., February 16, 1977.
10. Blue Cross to withdraw sensitive queries from form, *Psychiatric News,* July 1, 1977, pp. 1, 10, 16.
11. Altman, H. G.: Letter to the editor, "APA and FEP," *Psychiatric News,* August 19, 1977, p. 2.
12. APA, CHAMPUS enter claims criterion pact, *Psychiatric News,* August 19, 1977, pp. 1, 4.
13. Who can see CHAMPUS files? *Air Force Times,* July 23, 1979, p. 5.
14. Wedekind, L. H.: Your Medical Privacy *vs* the Services' Need to Know, *The Times Magazine,* March 5, 1979, pp. 7-11.
15. *Federal Register,* Vol. 43, No. 152, Monday, August 7, 1978, pp. 34958-34960; Ibid, April 4, 1977 re CHAMPUS: U.S. Code, Title 32, Sections 286, 286a, 286b, 297.
16. CHAMPUS continued focus of APA dispute. *Psychiatric News,* June 1, 1979, pp. 1, 4, 5.
17. APA objects to record access. *Psychiatric News,* June 1, 1979, pp. 1, 5.
18. PL 93-282, The Federal Alcohol and Drug Abuse Treatment Programs; 42 U.S. Code 4582, pp. 29-30; 40 *Federal Register* 27802 ff, July 1, 1975.
19. Public Law 95-142, October 25, 1977, 91 STAT 1189 Section 1166 (b) (1)-(5).
20. McMahon, G. and Beigler, J. S.: Minority Report submitted by the Committee on Confidentiality to the Committee on Health Insurance for Mental Disorders of the APA Board of Trustees regarding the meeting between the Commission on Standards of Practice and Third Party Payments and Representatives of the Department of Defense and CHAMPUS, March 5, 1979.
21. McMahon, G.: Summary report of the APA Committee on Confidentiality on the proposed CHAMPUS Peer Review Project, April, 1979, p. 5.
22. Assembly approves DSM-III, CHAMPUS Peer Review. *Psychiatric News,* June 15, 1979, pp. 1, 12.
23. Penner, N.: Letter to APA district branch presidents, June 27, 1979.
24. McGrath, J. J.: Letters to APA officers and to members of the Washington Psychiatric Society, July 30, 1979 and August 1, 1979 from the President of the WPS.
25. Kuder, A. U.: Letter to John J. McGrath, President, WPS, July 31, 1979.
26. Virginia Code, Title 37, Sections 37.1-225 — 37.1-226, 1978.
27. Personal communication from the December, 1979 meeting of the APA Commission on Professional Practices and Third Party Payments, New York, N.Y.

88   *Law and Ethics in the Practice of Psychiatry*

28. Kennison, W. S.: Presentation before the Legislative Issues Committee, American Psychoanalytic Association, Chicago, May 4, 1979.
29. Beigler, J. S.: The 1971 amendment of the Illinois statute on confidentiality: a new development in privilege law. *Amer. J. Psychiatry,* 129:311-315, 1972.
30. Linowes, D. F. (chairman): Personal Privacy in an Information Society. The Report of the Privacy Protection Study Commission. Washington, D.C., U.S. Government Printing Office, July 1977.
31. *Family Educational Rights and Privacy Act,* 20 U.S. Code 1232 g.
32. Justice Krever, H., Ontario, Canada, Supreme Court; head of Royal Commission of Inquiry into the Confidentiality of Health Records: Keynote Address: Privacy vs. Special Interests. Summarized in 6 pp. 2-7.
33. Official Actions of the American Psychiatric Association. Model law on confidentiality of health and social service records. *Amer. J. Psychiatry,* 136:138-147, 1979, Section 12, p. 142.
34. *District of Columbia Mental Health Information Act of 1978,* Title V, Section 501-504.
35. Spingarn, N. D. (Ed.): *Confidentiality: A Report of the 1974 Conference on Confidentiality of Health Records.* Washington, D.C. APA, 1975, pp. 8-20.
36. Official Actions of the American Psychiatric Association. Model law on confidentiality of health and social service records. *Amer. J. Psychiatry,* 136:138-147, 1979, Section 14, p. 142.
37. State of Illinois mental health and developmental disabilities confidentiality act. Springfield, State of Illinois Dept. of Mental Health and Developmental Disabilities, 1979, Section 3 (b).
38. *District of Columbia Mental Health Information Act of 1978,* Title I, Section 103.
39. Judge bars bid for doctor's file in trial of sex slayings suspect. *New York Times,* October 11, 1979, p. A9.
40. The Principles of Medical Ethics with Annotations especially Applicable to Psychiatry. Washington, D.C., Amer. Psychiatric Assn., Section 9, pp. 9-10.
41. *Doe v. Roe,* 345 N.Y.S. 2d 560, aff'd; 20 ALR 3d 1109.
42. Levin, T.: *Federal and State Judicial Decisions on Health Record Confidentiality.* Washington, D.C. National Commission on Confidentiality of Health Records, 1979.
43. *Horne v. Patton,* 291 Ala. 701, 287 So. 2d 824 (1973).
44. *Alexander v. Knight,* 197 Pa. Super. Ct. 79, 177 A — 2d 142 (1962).
45. *Felis v. Greenberg,* 51 Misc. 2d 441 273 N.Y.S. 2d 288 (Sup. Ct. 1966).
46. In re "B," 394 A. 2d 419 (Pa. 1978).
47. Beigler, J. S.: Psychiatric ethics and confidentiality. In Bloch, S. and Chodoff, P. (Eds.): *Psychiatric Ethics.* Oxford: Oxford University Press, in press.
48. In re Culbertson's Will, 57 Misc. 2d 391, 292 N.Y.S. 2d 806 (Sup. Ct. Erie Co. 1968).
49. Estate of Finkle, 395 N.Y.S. 2d 343 (N.Y.S. 1977).
50. Dole, V. P. and Nyswander, M. E.: Methadone maintenance treatment: A ten-year perspective. *J. Amer. Med. Assn.* 235:2117-2119, 1976.

51. Zane, M.: Suit filed over drug clinic raid. *San Francisco Chronicle*, August 29, 1979.

52. *Tarasoff vs. Regents of Univ of Cal.*, 529 P. 2d 55, 118 Cal. Rptr. 129 (1974) (Tarasoff I; 17 Cal. 3d 425, 551 P. 2d 334, 331 Cal. Rprtr. 14 (1976) (Tarasoff II).

53. Grossman, M.: Confidentiality: The right to privacy versus the right to know. In W. E. Barton and C. J. Sanborn (Eds.), *Law and the Mental Health Professions*. New York: International Universities Press, 1978, pp. 156-175.

54. *Nancy Schneider v. Vine Street Clinic et al.*, No. 78 L 16, Logan County, Illinois, 11th Circuit, December 7, 1978; Amicus brief No. 15344 in the Appellate Court of Illinois Fourth District, July, 1979.

55. *Peggy McIntosh v. Michael Milano, M.D.*, Supreme Court of New Jersey, Bergen County. Docket No. L-44368-76, Calendar No. 77-3811.

56. APA Committee on Confidentiality, recommended APA position statement on the Tarasoff decision, May, 1979.

57. Wise, T. P.: Where the public peril begins. A survey of psychotherapists to determine the effects of *Tarasoff*. *Stanford Law Review*, 31:165-190, 1978.

58. Gurevitz, H.: Unpublished survey, 1977.

59. *Zurcher v. Stanford Daily*, 46 LW 4546, U.S. Supreme Court, May 31, 1978.

60. Beigler, J. S. and Grossman, M.: *Hearings before the Subcommittee on the Constitution of the Committee on the Judiciary*, U.S. Senate, 95th Congress, second session on S. 3162, a bill to secure and protect the freedom of individuals from unwarranted intrusions by persons acting under color of law. Washington, D.C., U.S. Govt. Printing Office, 1979, pp. 223-277, p. 225.

61. Beigler, J. S.: Testimony of the APA before the Subcommittee on Courts, Civil Liberties and The Administration of Justice of the House Committee on the Judiciary, U.S. House of Representatives, on H.R. 3486 and the implications of *Zurcher v. Stanford Daily*, June 1, 1979.

62. Court stops state seizure of records. *Psychiatric News*, February 1, 1980, pp. 1, 33.

63. Cronkite, Walter: A supreme threat to freedom of press. *Chicago Sun-Times*, March 20, 1979, p. 33.

64. S. 3162, S. 3164, 95th Congress, 1978; H.R. 3486, 96th Congress, 1979.

65. Bar refuses to support curb on 'third party' searches. *New York Times*, August 10, 1979, p. A12.

66. Javits, J. *Congressional Record Proceedings and Debates of the 96th Congress*, first session: 125 No. 24, S1845-S1853, March 1, 1979.

67. Starting to protect privacy. Editorial. *N.Y. Times*, April 10, 1979.

68. Ribicoff, A.: S. 865 Privacy of Medical Information Act, pp. 3874-3882; S. 867 Privacy of Research Records Act, pp. 3883-3888, *Congressional Record*, 125, April 4, 1979.

69. Beigler, J. S.: Statement of the APA before the Subcommittee on Government Information and Individual Rights of the Committee on Government Operations, U.S. House of Representatives, April 9, 1979.

70. Goin, M.: Statement of the APA before the Governmental Affairs Com-

mittee, U.S. Senate, August 3, 1979; APA Confidentiality Chair appears before senate panel. *APA Legislative Newsletter,* August, 1979, p. 1.

71. Statement of the AMA to the Subcommittee on Government Information and Individual Rights, Committee on Government Operations, U.S. House of Representatives, Re: HR2979 and HR3444, December 7, 1979.

72. Lewis, T.: Protecting Privacy, *Am. Med. News,* March 7, 1980, pp. 3, 10.

73. Text of the President's State of the Union Address to a Joint Session of Congress, *N.Y. Times,* January 24, 1980, p. A12.

74. Congress Moves to Relax Curbs on CIA. *Science,* 207:965-966, 29 February, 1980.

75. Public Health Service, HEW, 42 CFR Part 2, Confidentiality of Alcohol and Drug Abuse Patient Records, *Federal Register,* 45: No. 1, Wednesday, January 2, 1980, pp. 53-54.

76. Bloch, S.: Letter to the Editor: Soviet Psychiatry, *Psychiatric News,* February 15, 1980, pp. 2, 8.

77. Cited by Linowes, D. F.: Must personal privacy die in the computer age? *Amer. Bar Assn. Journal,* 65:1180-1184, August, 1979, p. 1184.

4

Disclosure and Consent in Psychiatric Practice: Mission Impossible?

Jay Katz, M.D.

The discovery of a new world in which people live by the rule of informed consent is still far off. If indeed such a world exists on some distant shore, one must first traverse uncharted waters, sail through treacherous currents, and navigate between Scylla and Charybdis. If readers feel, after having perused this essay, that I have taken them on such a journey without sighting land, they will have understood me well. Many intricate problems need to be better understood before the idea of informed consent can guide the interactions between patients and their psychiatrists. That it cannot do so now will become abundantly clear.

It would serve little purpose, and ultimately would only add to the confusion, if I were to discuss the law of informed consent

The financial support of the Commonwealth Foundation and the Kayden Foundation is gratefully acknowledged.

as it applies, for example, to voluntary and involuntary commitment proceedings or to the administration of drugs, electroconvulsive treatments, and psychotherapy. To do justice to such an approach would require a careful examination of each court opinion on each topic; for, more likely than not, the opinions will prove to be internally inconsistent, in conflict with other decisions, and subject to challenge when the next similar case arises. Any conclusions one might reach about the state of the law would have to be tempered by qualifications as to their applicability to other fact situations. Moreover, the many reservations which psychiatrists might have regarding the significance of each decision for professional practice would have to be addressed. Drawing conclusions would be a tedious task and, more importantly, distract from the appreciation of the more fundamental underlying problems which professionals and judges need to understand better prior to an examination of case law and prior to the writing of the next opinion. I prefer, and I believe it is more in keeping with the ethos of the American College of Psychiatrists, to explicate the complexities of informed consent by presenting my analysis of the idea of informed consent as it is seen through the eyes of the legal, medical and psychiatric professions.

I should make it clear at the outset that the *doctrine* of informed consent must be distinguished from the *idea* of informed consent. The former reflects the legal profession's responses—albeit ambivalent, conflicting, and limited—to the perceived need for greater communication between doctors and patients. The latter speaks to the quest for a doctrine which takes informed consent seriously by first asking: What factors need to be better understood before one can have a doctrine which grants patients the right to participate in the medical decision-making process? Thus, when I speak of the idea of informed consent, I have only this quest in mind. The duties and obligations which fidelity to the idea of informed consent will impose on both parties, should the search continue, remain to be seen. In today's world, it is by and large a charade.

LAW'S VISION

The doctrine of informed consent surfaced in case law only 23 years ago in *Salgo v. Leland Stanford, Jr. University Board of Trustees* (1). Justice Bray introduced it, in almost *deus ex machina* fashion, at the end of the *Salgo* opinion in a brief paragraph. He commanded physicians "in discussing the element of risk [to employ] a certain amount of *discretion* consistent with the *full disclosure* of facts necessary to an informed consent" (2). The juxtaposition of discretion and full disclosure was a startling piece of judicial work. Clearly, informed consent was born in confusion.

For years, I searched for informed consent's roots. Extensive research revealed no antecedent cases, and I only discovered its true parents when I examined the briefs submitted to the California Court of Appeals. The entire paragraph set forth in Justice Bray's opinion had been copied from the amicus brief of the American College of Surgeons (3). Is it not an ironic twist of history that informed consent, so bitterly opposed by most physicians, was dreamed up by lawyers in the employ of doctors?

The American College of Surgeons and their lawyers probably composed that paragraph for reasons similar to those which three years later led Justice Schroeder of the Kansas Supreme Court, in *Natanson v. Kline* (4), to adopt the language of *Salgo* and to write the first comprehensive opinion on informed consent, which shaped malpractice law in most American jurisdictions for the next decade. Neither Mr. Salgo nor Mrs. Natanson were told anything about the risks of the newly introduced medical procedures they had been asked to undergo. It was this *total* silence which disturbed physicians, lawyers, and judges alike. Why it took such a long time to appreciate that there was something wrong with leaving patients so completely in the dark about diagnostic procedures and therapeutic interventions is an intriguing question, and so is the question as to why two judges suddenly challenged such omissions in the late 1950s. After all, prior to 1957, many cases with similar fact situations had been litigated and decided in favor of physician-defendants. Most likely a number of factors converged: a greater consciousness of the rights of citizen-patients to make their own decisions; an increasing awareness that the spectacular advances in medical technology not only bestowed benefits but also created their own formidable and uncontrollable risks; the employment of such new and powerful interventions in *Salgo* and *Natanson;* and the total absence of any risk disclosure in both instances.

Justice Schroeder opened his opinion with a powerful appeal to fundamental jurisprudential principles:

> Anglo-American law starts with the premise of thorough-going self-determination. It follows that each man is considered to be master of his own body, and he may, if he be of sound mind, expressly prohibit the performance of life-saving surgery, or other medical treatment. A doctor might well believe that an operation or form of treatment is desirable or necessary but the law does not permit him to substitute his own judgment for that of the patient by any form of artifice or deception (5).

These principles, however, must be placed in context, for Justice Schroeder surrounded them with qualifications which robbed them of their force. Most crucial were his adoptions of: 1) the "reasonable and prudent medical doctor" standard, limiting disclosure to what physicians in the community would commonly reveal (6), and 2) the therapeutic privilege exception which permits physicians to withhold information whenever disclosure "would seriously jeopardize the recovery of an unstable, temperamental or severely depressed patient" (7). Since physicians are generally not committed to patients' participation in the medical decision-making process, the first qualification in particular stifled Justice Schroeder's call for self-determination.

Neither the *Natanson* court, nor 12 years later the *Canterbury* (8) and *Cobbs* (9) courts, despite the latters' substitution of "a standard set by law" for the reasonable medical doctor standard, were willing to assert that whenever lack of disclosure vitiates whatever consent had been given, liability should be established under stringent trespass doctrines instead of the more lenient negligence law. The law of trespass evolved to protect citizens against unauthorized invasions and to provide remedies for the indignity of unconsented interventions. The law of negligence, on the other hand, has always favored physicians over patients, and while this posture may have merit in situations of negligence, different considerations apply under trespass. In the case of trespass law, it should not matter, for example, whether or not the patient suffered any physical injuries. Principles of "thoroughgoing self-determination" and pronouncements that "the consent to what happens to one's self is the informed exercise of a choice" should have led judges to impose liability for any intervention which did not comport with these principled assertions. Instead Judge Robinson invoked the rule of negligence when he settled the matter of *Canterbury*:

> No more than breach of any other legal duty does non-fulfillment of the physician's obligation to disclose alone establish liability to the patient. An unrevealed risk must materialize, for otherwise the omission, *however unpardonable,* is legally without consequence (10).

Other purposes of tort law may have required such a resolution.

Viewed from the vantage point of patients' autonomy, however, the case law on informed consent raises serious questions about courts' thorough-going commitment to self-determination. This shaky commitment extends to juries and legislatures. When *Canterbury* and *Cobbs* were retried, the juries returned verdicts in favor of defendant-physicians. And recently a number of legislatures have passed informed consent statutes which greatly limit the doctrine's scope (11). Georgia abolished informed consent altogether (12). One judge expressed a not unusual viewpoint succinctly, "children play at the game of being a doctor, but judges and juries ought not" (13).

I have documented elsewhere judges' weak commitment to the doctrine of informed consent (14). Although Anglo-American jurisprudential theories forced its promulgation, judges, once they attempted to construe it, began to appreciate the problems implementation posed and they retreated. What has emerged is a hodgepodge of appeals to "thorough-going self-determination" and deference to professional paternalism.

Judges, because they are aware of the fact that most of what takes place in medical practice is beyond their expertise, have generally been reluctant to regulate the physician-patient relationship. Even though informed consent raised issues with which they were familiar, they listened to physicians who asserted forcefully that patients are too ignorant to make decisions on their own behalf, that disclosure increases patients' fears and reinforces foolish decisions, and that informing them about the uncertainties of medical interventions in many instances seriously undermines the faith which is so essential to the success of therapy. Judges did not probe these contentions in depth and were persuaded to refrain from interfering significantly with traditional medical practices.

Judges' reluctance to break new ground was aided and abetted by their own ambivalence about whether physicians or patients are the more appropriate decision-makers. Though judges understood that this problem had to be considered from the viewpoints of both professionals *and* patients, the tensions engendered by conflicting wishes to defer to professional practices and to respect citizen-patient decision-making ultimately proved too difficult to reconcile. Being professionals themselves, judges identified more readily with fellow professionals. This identification was made easier by giving considerable weight to physicians' "rational" commitment to placing patients' physical well-being and longevity above all else, and contrasting this commitment with the often-made claim that patients tended to make "irrational" and "foolish" decisions. The concern over patients' alleged incapacity for rational choice probably was the most important determinant in not jarring too much the cakes of custom. In doing so, courts ignored the fact that consent and the idea of informed consent are embedded in the legal principle of personal freedom.

The legal doctrine of informed consent does not significantly advance patients' right to meaningful participation in the medical decision-making process. It merely places a new duty upon physicians to recite the risks of any intervention they propose and perhaps, though this issue is by no means settled, to inform patients of alternative treatments. Thus, after all is said and done, informed consent merely imposes a duty to deliver a disclosure monologue. Disclosure alone, however, does little to expand opportunities for meaningful consent, particularly in surrender-prone medical settings. To achieve that objective, patients' rights and needs to participate in medical decisions affecting their lives must be accorded greater respect.

Commentators in general and physicians in particular have insufficiently appreciated law's confused and limited vision of informed consent. The doctrine gives physicians great latitude to practice medicine as they have always done, as long as they are now prepared to recite some of the risks of the proposed intervention. Thus, the countless professional articles and editorials which excoriate law for the imposition of onerous obligations are beside the point. They attribute to law a broader vision of informed consent than exists.

MEDICINE'S VISION

Physicians' reactions to informed consent still puzzle me. I am not surprised by the adamant negative response or by the fact that little has changed, rhetoric notwithstanding, with respect to patients' participation in decision-making. Good reasons—which I shall shortly address—can be advanced for such attitudes. What surprises me is the acknowledgment by professionals, in the midst of all kinds of reservations and opposition, that patients are entitled to know "something." Although the "something" is never precisely identified, I have begun to ask myself: Why this grudging admission? After all, secrecy is deeply embedded in the Hippocratic tradition: "I will impart a knowledge of the Art to my own sons . . . teachers [and] disciples . . . but to none others" (15). Or put more directly by Hippocrates in his admonitions to physicians:

> Perform [these duties] calmly and adroitly, concealing most things from the patient while you are attending to him. Give necessary orders with cheerfulness and sincerity, turning his

attention away from what is being done to him; sometimes reprove sharply and empathically, and sometimes comfort with solicitude and attention, revealing nothing of the patient's future or present condition . . . (16).

One explanation has occurred to me. The advent of scientific medicine may have engendered conflicting tensions between Hippocratic secrecy and the scientific ethos of sharing discoveries and knowledge from which the patient could, in theory, not easily be excluded. In practice, however, little has changed; for whatever disquiet the exclusion of patients created was quickly silenced by the conviction that patients are too uneducated to understand "esoteric knowledge" (17). These tensions are compounded in the practice of psychiatry for an additional reason. Dynamic psychiatry champions openness of dialogue between psychiatrist and patient. But that commitment too was short-circuited by limiting disclosure to information which psychiatrists consider therapeutic. The idea of informed consent was not powerful enough to make much headway against these overwhelming odds.

Whatever the contemporary tensions, clearly medicine throughout its history has never taken any affirmative position on the duty of physicians to inform or even to converse with patients. The Hippocratic Oath makes no references to such an obligation, nor do the *Principles of Medical Ethics* of the American Medical Association (18). Parsons' writings on the medical profession, which have profoundly influenced contemporary thought on physician-patient interactions, support the Hippocratic tradition. Parsons insists that patients must trustingly and unquestioningly place themselves in doctors' hands. Patients "must take [physicians'] judgments and measures on 'authority'. . . . We often speak of 'doctor's orders' " (19).

Clearly disclosure and consent, for purposes of inviting patients to participate in decision-making, have no historical roots in medical practice. Before proposing any departure from existing practice, one must pause and ponder this remarkable fact and ask: What is it about medical practice which invited such an unwavering historical development? Consider MacIntyre's observations:

> Traditionally, the patient puts himself in the doctor's hand. The doctor generally in return does not advise the patient of a variety of possibilities and leaves the patient to decide; he generally does not in fact reveal to the patient his own processes of thinking. . . . Instead he *tells* the patient what is necessary. . . . In our culture only this kind of medical authority does not appear to us as odd and singular as it is, because we are familiarized with it from early childhood; but when we do learn to notice it, its oddity is all the more obtrusive because it is so very nearly without parallel in the rest of our social experience (20).

I believe MacIntyre is wrong in asserting that medical behavior is "without parallel." The behavior is not limited to medicine alone; it extends to the practices of all professions. More important, MacIntyre does not entertain the possibility that the behavior he questions may express not only doctors' proclivities for giving orders but also patients' propensities for receiving orders. Thus the "oddity" which puzzles him may say something profound about human needs to give and follow orders, in general, and about human capacities to inform and be informed, in particular.

Before turning to these issues, I can only note in passing that any change in professional values and belief systems is a slow process. Therefore, it would be surprising, indeed suspect, if the recent interest in disclosure and consent had already made a significant impact on existing practices. Pertinent here are Freud's comments on the stability of the superego, which constitutes "the vehicle of tradition and of all time-resisting judgments of value which have propagated themselves in this manner from generation to generation. . . . Mankind never lives entirely in the present. The past, the tradition of the race and of the professions live on in the ideologies of the superego, and yield only slowly to the influences of the present and to new changes . . ." (21). Any call for greater patient participation in decision-making has to take into account the historical reality of physician-patient interactions and the residues left behind in the consciences of professionals, which, in turn, are transmitted during each generation from teacher to student.

If my analysis of law's limited response to and medicine's inexperience with disclosure and consent is correct, one should resist being seduced by the rhetoric that the last two decades have wrought fundamental change in physician-patient interactions. Such siren calls deceive. Doctors' orders, on the one hand, and passive acquiescence, silent noncompliance, or stubborn refusal, on the other, rather than dialogue, continue to govern the relations between physicians and patients.

I hope that my observations of law's and medicine's vision are not perceived as an indictment of judges and doctors. As patients have taught us, the identifying of conflicts and their defensive and adaptive implications are often heard as putdowns. My rather blunt remarks are intended not to indict, but to impress upon the reader that the life of informed consent will not be an easy one when, and if, it ever comes to pass. It is the premature announcement of the birth of a sturdy infant which has created confusion, and it is the confusion to which I wanted to call attention.

PSYCHIATRY'S VISION

My inquiry into disclosure and consent has led me to appreciate that much of psychiatry's discontent with the state of its art and science, particularly in its therapeutic practices, cannot be assuaged by embracing the medical model; for psychiatry and medicine share similar fundamental problems in that both are plagued by the spectre of uncertainty. As Feinstein so forcefully noted:

> Radical surgery and irradiation therapy in cancer have both been available for more than 60 years, but their therapeutic contributions in many neoplasms remain obscure and controversial. Although anticoagulants, antibiotics, hypotensive agents, insulin, and steroids have been available for 15 to 40 years, many of their true effects on patients and diseases are unknown or equivocal. Clinicians are still uncertain about the best means of treatment for even such routine problems

as a common cold, a stroke, a myocardial infarction, an obstetrical delivery, or an acute psychotic depression. . . . At a time of potent drugs and formidable surgery, the exact effects of many therapeutic procedures are dubious and shrouded in dissension—often documented either by the unquantified data of "experience" or by grandiose statistics whose mathematical formulations are so clinically naive that any significance is purely numerical rather than biologic (22).

I offer Feinstein's observations not to provide solace but to underscore my belief that a greater awareness of the uncertainty which haunts psychiatric practices is essential before any meaningful prescriptions for disclosure and consent can be provided.

Consider, for example, the many treatment options available in psychiatric practice: individual psychotherapy, group psychotherapy, biofeedback, psychoanalysis, chemotherapy, family therapy, psychosurgery, encounter groups, electroconvulsive treatment, behavior modifications, sex therapy, self-help therapy, and so on. Add to the complexities introduced by this fact alone, the variations in technique employed by individual psychiatrists in the practice of each of these therapies which have a profound and unknown impact on therapeutic outcome. Add to this the lack of consensus on the effectiveness of any of these treatments, and the far-reaching, though still unclear, implications of offering patients supposedly suppressive, conditioning, supportive, or self-understanding therapies. Psychiatrists are aware of these uncertainties; they are discussed in their meetings and journals. Yet in the consulting room, in their discussions with patients, certainty rather than uncertainty reigns, infecting psychiatrist and patient alike.

Psychiatry is under heavy attack for the lack of data on the effectiveness of its therapies (23). The question—"Does psychotherapy work "—is being raised within the profession, in Congress, by insurance companies, and in many other quarters. It is an uncomfortable question because psychiatrists can provide few answers supported by hard data. Psychiatrists, however, are not alone in facing this question. Does tonsillectomy, coronary bypass surgery, hysterectomy, or chemotherapy work? The medical model, except in a few isolated instances, has not supplied satisfactory answers on effectiveness either.

Before commenting on the implications of these and other uncertainties for informed consent, I should pause and all too briefly indicate what I mean by uncertainty. What follows is quite tentative for I have not yet sorted out to my satisfaction how to best present the issues which concern me. Uncertainty, like the head of the god Janus, points in two different directions. First, there are the uncertainties engendered by the inadequate and incomplete knowledge which informs the art and science of medicine, and of psychiatry as well. Feinstein's and my illustrations make abundantly clear that this uncertainty is vast. Many of these uncertainties, if one has perspicacity and courage, can be consciously confronted. But there is a second kind of uncertainty of equally vast proportion, which expresses itself in a false sense of certainty. What I have in mind is the substitution of certainty for uncertainty which is engendered by an unawareness that existing knowledge has been insufficiently mastered, or by unexamined assumptions, unexamined value choices, and unexamined personal convictions. Many of these uncertainties are unconscious, though some of them could rise to consciousness if individuals attended to them.

I place both kinds of uncertainty under the same rubric because their impact on physician-patient communication, unless great care is taken, is equally great. Since uncertainties of the first type (i.e., those resulting from the state of inadequate knowledge) make it more difficult, for example, to distinguish between convictions based on fact and those based on value judgment, the two types of uncertainty reinforce one another and preclude making clear distinctions between the two in practice.

The uncertainties I have described and their impact on psychiatrists and patients challenge the implementation of the idea of informed consent. Many questions about the feasibility of informing patients must first be posed and answered. Consider, for example, the range of treatment options available to patients. Inasmuch as a decision in favor of one form of psychiatric therapy over another represents a combination of medical, emotional, aesthetic, religious, philosophical, social, interpersonal, and personal judgments, can these judgments be sorted out? If they can be, which of these component judgments should be made by the psychiatrist and which by the patient? In the light of the uncertainties about efficacy, what information can and should be shared with patients prior to embarking on a voyage into the unknown?

These questions lead to even more fundamental ones: Is it possible for psychiatrists to inform and for patients to be informed about the choices available to them? Can psychiatrists become more aware of their proclivity to substitute certainty for uncertainty? Which of their uncertainties should they share with patients? What are the consequences of such sharing? Can patients tolerate awareness of uncertainty, so necessary for giving meaningful consent? These are important questions, which, though difficult to answer, must be confronted in order to define the limits of informed consent in guiding decision-making between psychiatrists and patients.

The proclivity to substitute certainty for uncertainty is probably a universal human tendency, which serves both adaptive and defensive needs. Psychiatrists, therefore, are uniquely qualified to make a contribution to the understanding of this impediment to informed consent. In what follows I shall focus on the all too vague notions of what constitutes competence and autonomy as well as of the ways in which both are affected by transference, countertransference, and regression phenomena.

Competence

Psychiatrists and lawyers have been engaged in an acrimonious debate over the ambit of competence. That debate, to its detriment, has focused on supposed disagreements over the psychological nature of human beings in general or of offenders in particular. The two professions, I believe, are not too far apart on that theoretical issue; what separates them are differing views on a more practical question: To what extent can or should law and society take psychological considerations into account in the administration of "justice"? Personal responsibility, which rests so much on human capacities to be in touch with the interplay of conscious and unconscious dynamisms, is tricky to determine anywhere, and particularly in a court of law.

Since psychiatrists encounter patients who range from the normally competent to the grossly incompetent, let me make a few remarks about incompetence before addressing competence. Most psychiatrists, I am sure, agree that competent and incompetent functioning cannot be neatly assessed. It is always a question of more or less, of one *and* the other, aggravated and attenuated by internal and external factors. Since external factors affect the balance between competence and incompetence, and do so to significantly differing degrees, the question must always be posed: incompetent for what external purposes? Here I need only address the question of incompetence for making decisions about treatment. In these situations, psychiatrists might, as is true in law, presume competence and only in rare and well-specified circumstances seek authorization to override their patients' wishes. I realize that such a radical shift in professional attitudes may preclude treatment for persons in need of treatment and this is sad. Yet a price has to be paid in adopting one policy over another.

One assumption which underlies the presumption of incompetence has always concerned me. Physicians in general and psychiatrists in particular have been guided all too unquestioningly by the belief that they are the guardians of the health of all citizens rather than only of those who agree to place themselves in their care. This conviction has compromised the dialogue between psychiatrists and their prospective patients. Any doubts about treatment on the part of persons not yet patients are all too thoughtlessly interpreted as a confirmation that there is something wrong with them. The option of no treatment, whenever it is implicitly or explicitly in patients' minds, cannot be explored, and they are dispatched instead to a Procrustean couch. The presumption of competence will improve the dialogue, indeed it will create for the first time a climate for dialogue. What passes for dialogue in today's world is instead a monologue, delivered to patients who are there to be seen but not to be heard.

If professionals viewed the desirability of treatment both from their own and their patients' perspective, it might become easier to identify those who need care despite protests to the contrary and to promulgate safeguards for preventing abuse of such awesome authority. Moreover, a presumption of competence would alert psychiatrists not to fall victim to the temptation of listening with a third ear for manifestations of the irrational, so appropriate for therapeutic purposes but not necessarily for decisional ones.

What I have in mind is illustrated by a recent Massachusetts decision, *Rogers v. Okin* (24). Judge Tauro ruled that hospitalized mental patients, except in emergencies, have the constitutional right to refuse treatment. Dr. Alan Stone, then president of the American Psychiatric Association, called it "probably the most impossible, ill-considered judicial decision in the field of mental health law" (25). I do not wish to debate whether or not this is a correct assessment. I can, however, understand why Judge Tauro felt compelled to write his opinion. Throughout the proceedings, the defendant-psychiatrists maintained that "a committed mental patient is *per se* incompetent to decide whether or not to receive treatment" (26), that "once an individual becomes incompetent . . . the duty and right [exist] to care for the 'best interest' of the incompetent" (27), that "a sincere [professional] belief . . . that such treatment is necessary to the patient's recovery" (28) should be respected, and that even voluntary patients "may not second-guess the institution staff by picking and choosing the type of medication to be used" (29). Such authority is too sweeping and, if granted, would preclude any possibility of dialogue between psychiatrist and patients.

As my colleague Robert A. Burt has warned repeatedly in his recent book, *Taking Care of Strangers*, "assigning exclusive choice-making authority in one party (whether patient, physician, or judge) and complementary choiceless status to another in an interpersonal transaction readily leads to paradoxically destructive results for all participants" (30). It is this warning which the defendant-psychiatrists did not hear or at least did not heed. If they had, they might have been moved to define most narrowly the situations in which they wanted the State to authorize their exercising such awesome power. Their assertions made it easier for Judge Tauro to counter:

> The only purpose of forced medication, in a non-emergency, is to help the patient. The desire to help the patient is a laudable if not noble goal. But, a basic premise of the right to privacy is the freedom to decide whether we want to be left alone. It takes a grave set of circumstances to abrogate the right. That a non-emergency injection in the buttocks may be therapeutic does not constitute such a circumstance. . . .
>
> There are alternative methods of treating mental patients, though some may be slower and less effective than psychotropic medication. Plaintiff's primary objection is to the forced injection of psychotropic medication. Given the alternatives available in non-emergencies, subjecting a patient to the humiliation of being disrobed and then injected with drugs powerful enough to immobilize both body and mind is totally unreasonable by any standard (31).

I had promised no cases. But this case, which came to my attention only after I was well into writing this chapter and which will send psychiatrists and lawyers into the trenches once again, calls for some comments. I am not saying that *Rogers v. Okin* is either a good or bad opinion, I am only saying that psychiatrists deserve such opinions as long as they ask for such exclusive and indiscriminate choice-making authority.

Psychiatrists' doubts about the capacity of their patients to make decisions on their own behalf, however, extend not only to "incompetent" persons but to competent ones as well. Indeed the fuzzy line between incompetence and competence, as *Rogers v. Okin* illustrates, contributes to these doubts. What has been overlooked is that competence is not a fixed personality characteristic. The context in which it is evaluated has a significant impact on the conclusions reached. Moreover, transference, countertransference, and regression powerfully affect its evaluation. It is to these phenomena I now turn and what follows will raise profound questions about human beings' capacity to inform and be informed. At the same time, I shall argue that the concepts of transference, countertransference and regression have also been employed, however unwittingly, in the service of viewing patients as less competent than they actually are. If I am correct, then change is possible, and it is the extent of possible change which will ultimately define the limits of the idea of informed consent. In the absence of any change, the idea of informed consent will remain the puppet show it is today.

Transference

The literature on transference is immense. It has illuminated much about the conflicting expectations which patients bring to therapeutic encounters. At the same time, much injustice has been done to persons and patients in the name of transference. To be sure, all human beings bring to their encounters with others the precipitates of early experiences. Such experiences, intensified during illness, during protracted contacts in the psychiatrist's office, or during any periods of emotional upheaval, shape a person's interactions with others in significant ways. But these very transferences express an important facet of an individual's uniqueness and essence, his/her personality, who he/she has become. Transferences—and this is often not kept in mind— are not necessarily pathological. They can, of course, misguide persons, particularly in times of stress and in encounters with persons who care for those under stress. This is a danger, but an equally great, perhaps even greater, danger is that caretakers have the power to manipulate and exploit transferences. It is this danger, insufficiently considered in the professional literature, which puts professionals to a crucial test: to do their utmost to withstand the temptation of exploiting their exalted position.

The problems, however, go deeper. The affirmation of transference has wittingly and unwittingly reinforced the traditional professional view that patients are indeed incompetent. Now, in addition to being seen as lacking expert knowledge, they are also viewed as bringing to their encounters with professionals irrational precipitates of their past, an incapacity to distinguish between childhood and present. Therefore, it is said, that they should not be trusted to make decisions on their own behalf.

Yet transference could teach us different lessons: to be aware of its ubiquitous presence and to address it in new ways. After all, psychiatrists since the days of Freud have been taught to interpret transference for therapeutic purposes. Now they also need to learn how to address transference manifestations for purposes of the decision-making dialogue with patients. This may prove less problematic in patients' encounters with non-psychiatric physicians, although the latter have woefully, however unwittingly, exploited transference phenomena. The history of the placebo effect (32) speaks eloquently to that fact.

Since the proper management of the long-term psychotherapeutic process may require not commenting prematurely on emerging transference manifestations, doing so for purposes of decision-making may create new problems. They may, however, be not as insurmountable as first appearances suggest. While it has often been asserted that the distinction between diagnostic and therapeutic encounters makes little sense—in other words, that therapy begins from the moment a patient first enters a psychiatrist's office—the uncritical embrace of such assertions can do violence to the person, not yet a patient, as a choice-making individual. The premature professional commitment to treatment, fed by prospective patients' transference readiness, may short-circuit any discussion of patients' view on the need for treatment and the choice of treatment. Agreement and abject surrender imperceptibly blend, and whatever happens subsequently is affected by the fact that it was the doctor's judgment, and not necessarily the patient's, which led to treatment. The idea of informed consent illuminates here something crucial, which has generally gone awry in the initial interviews between psychiatrists and patients. All kinds of unnoticed coercions, however much informed by the scientific convictions of the therapist, become a part of the conversation between psychiatrist and patient. Such coercions often come to haunt subsequent treatment. What then is labelled as resistance is often more than just that; it may also be a reaction to having been seduced into following doctors' orders in the first place.

If psychiatric treatment is to be based on shared objectives, it requires shared decision-making about treatment. I believe that many patients, if the opportunities are provided, can and will participate in decision-making. Providing such opportunities will create a much better climate for the entire therapeutic process than exists in contemporary practice. My prescriptions, however, need to be evaluated against the capacities of both professionals and patients to address the uncertainties inherent in psychiatric practices, as well as against the role of faith (33) as a significant ingredient in therapeutic effectiveness. I have in mind again, among other things, the placebo effect, i.e., that therapeutic effectiveness depends so much on the faith a doctor has in his therapy and, in turn, on the faith patients have in their doctor and his prescriptions (34).

Countertransference

It is striking, if one consults the literature on countertransference, how little has been written on that subject as compared to transference. In reading the few articles that do exist, one is also struck by the frequency with which countertransferences are defined primarily as those reactions in the therapist engendered *by* the patient. It is the patient who is identified as a prime mover of what is unleashed in the therapist. Always the patient!

There is, however, more to countertransference. The longer I reflect upon informed consent, the more convinced I become that professionals' countertransferences are a greater impediment to its meaningful implementation than patients' transferences. Roy Menninger understands this well:

> . . . the doctor has too much narcissistic investment in his power position vis-à-vis the patient. Many of us have developed subtle but disguised ways of maintaining that power position, all in the name of "good treatment." The fact is that medicine, as many of us practice it, encourages a patient's dependency. It does not encourage a more desirable

goal, namely the establishment of a kind of parity in the
relationship that promotes a greater responsibility by the
patient for his own treatment . . . Physicians generally do
not give enough attention to the need for enabling, encouraging, promoting patients to establish a greater sense of
individual control, a sense of mastery, through a kind of
therapeutic alliance rather than a therapeutic autocracy that
is psychologically and economically gratifying to the physician. I am well aware that our patients are expert at putting
us in a position narcissistically satisfying to us, making it
thereby more difficult to recognize this problem and to
change it . . . (35).

Consider, on the other hand, the implications of a diametrically
different view advanced by Brian Bird in his book, *Talking with
Patients*:

. . . Talking with patients, like the whole business of being
a doctor, is a very large order. Just how big, and just what
it all consists of, no one really knows.

One little understood thing that distinguishes being a doctor
from not being one is the position a doctor assumes relative
to people who come to him for help. The doctor's way of
responding to requests for help is his special thing; it is a
quality that transcends knowledge, a quality that demands
a unique sense of responsibility for human life, a responsibility built on an almost arrogant kind of confidence in
himself, a quality that has evolved from the age-old tradition
of patient care.

. . . he must accept within himself the seemingly arrogant
idea that he has the power, the right, the authority to do the
unusual, peculiar things "being a doctor" demands of him
. . . This final authority must come from him; he must have
the nerve, the confidence, the gall, or whatever it takes, to
grant it unto himself.

. . . Ordinary people do ordinary things, Only extraordinary
people do extraordinary things. It is in this sense that doctors
are indeed special. They are special, not because they are
more intelligent, more capable, more trustworthy, or more
anything else, but because the public has given them this
extraordinary role and they have accepted it . . . (36).

The title of the book is misleading. Talking *with* patients is impossible if the qualities Bird ascribes to physicians continue to rule the interactions between them and their patients. "The power, the right, the authority" he delegates to physicians will shape their professional personalities and affect in decisive ways their relationships with patients. Such attitudes are facets of countertransference phenomena which, since they are deeply ingrained in the ethos of professionalism and thus considered non-neurotic, have generally not been subsumed under that term. They should be, however, because they influence not only the initial dialogue with patients but also the entire treatment process to a hitherto unrecognized extent.

Countertransference, conceived as broadly as I suggest, would move to center stage the examination of the impact on psychiatrist-patient interactions of Aesculapian authority, of scientific value judgments, of personal beliefs, of the ways professionals deal with scientific and personal uncertainties, of attitudes toward patients, of how decisions ought to be made and of much more. Embarking on such an exploration will prove to be a rough journey; for psychiatrists have not been accustomed to looking that deeply into their professional and individual psyche; to look at our neurotic blind spots, as Freud prescribed, was hard enough.

Regression

It has long been known that the stress of illness leads to psychological regression, to chronologically earlier modes of functioning. What has been insufficiently explored, however, are the contributions which physicians' attitudes toward their patients make to that regressive pull; nor has much attention been paid to learning whether the regression can be reversed by not keeping patients in the dark, by inviting them to participate in decision-making, by addressing and nurturing the intact, mature parts of their functioning. Psychiatrists must explore this uncharted territory and learn what strains will be imposed on physicians and patients alike, if Anna Freud's admonition to students at the Case-Western Reserve Medical School are heeded:

. . . you must not be tempted to treat [the patient] as a child. You must be tolerant toward him as you would be toward a child and as respectful as you would be towards a fellow adult because he has only gone back to childhood as far as he's ill. He also has another part of his personality, which has remained intact and that part of him will resent it deeply, if you make too much of your authority . . . (37).

Professionals ask patients to be obedient and to follow doctor's orders. When such prescriptions turn them into children, submissive or obstreperous ones, the contributions which the disease, the physician, the patient or all three make to the regression are not given separate attention.

To return once more to competence. It has been insufficiently recognized that Hippocratic medical practices contribute to making patients appear and act more incompetent than they actually are. The traditional pattern of physician-patient interactions makes imcompetence a self-fulfilling prophesy.

Autonomy

The call for meaningful consent confronts the question of the patient's capacity for autonomous choice. In challenging such capacity, much has been made of the silent influence of self-destructive unconscious motivations, the quest for magical solutions, the regression to childhood behavior in the presence of illness, the strength of wishful thinking, the propensity to prefer immediate gratifications over more realistic future-oriented goals, and so forth. There is, of course, truth in these assertions but too much has been made of them. Embracing them totally could strip all patients, and nonpatients as well, of decision-making authority.

All human conduct is shaped by both conscious and unconscious motivations, reflective and unreflective thought, distorted and undistorted memories, attainable and unattainable aspirations, perceptions which take or do not take reality into account, impulses which brook no delay and those which can first be subjected to experimental thought. Autonomy—and this is the human dilemma—is never absolute; it is relative, and this truth holds for professionals and patients alike.

A lesson to be learned is that autonomy can never be taken for granted. Autonomy requires nurture and care, which communication and dialogue can provide by bringing into awareness all kinds of acknowledged and unconsidered influences on the choices about to be made. Thus, in professional-patient interactions, respect for patients' autonomy demands that patients be given sufficient information and that misconceptions and distortions which may affect their decisions be identified and clarified.

In their dialogue with patients, professionals should spare no effort to maximize patients' autonomy. Particularly in the face of patients' doubts or disagreements, psychiatrists should try as best they can both to understand their patients' objections and to make themselves understood. Therefore, psychiatrists' insistence that they and their patients converse and think together should be honored, even if patients initially resist such interactions. That much invasion of privacy must be tolerated in order to safeguard patients' autonomy through insight and not to allow it to be undermined by unnecessary fears, blind misconceptions, and false certainties. John Stuart Mill appreciated this: "Considerations to aid his judgment, exhortations to strengthen his will may be offered to him, even obtruded on him by others; but he himself is the final judge" (38). I realize that a recommendation of a possibly forced dialogue creates new dangers of overreaching and compulsion. But in insisting on conversation, I have in mind that the psychiatrist interact with the patient in the spirit of Leonardo da Vinci's distinctions between painting and sculpturing (39). In sculpturing—*per via di levare*—the figure comes into being by chiselling away "the distortions" introduced by the material; in painting—*per via di porre*—the painter adds his own "distortions" to the canvas. Thus, the psychiatrist must take great care to work with the patient's distortions without adding his own to them. The age-old controversy over autonomy can now be examined from a different perspective: respectful dialogue, which underlies the idea of informed consent, can nurture and extend autonomy—the psychiatrist's as well as the patient's.

CONCLUSION

Formidable barriers stand in the way of a meaningful decision-making dialogue between psychiatrists and patients. Whether, and the extent to which, these barriers should and could be removed ultimately depends on an answer to the question: Are psychiatrists *and* patients willing and able to collaborate in decision-making? The question does not readily yield an answer. All human beings, especially those who need and who give care, struggle with impulses both to maintain and to surrender their autonomy, often without being conscious that such contradictory wishes exist. And judges, professionals and patients bring to this dilemma profound doubts as to whether people are better served by siding with Dostoyevsky's Grand Inquisitor:

> And look what you have done . . . in the name of freedom! I tell you man has no more agonizing anxiety than to find someone to whom he can hand over with all speed the gift of freedom with which the unhappy creature is born . . . We have corrected your great work and have based it on miracle, mystery and authority. And men rejoiced that they were once more led like sheep and that the terrible gift [of freedom] which had brought them so much suffering had at last been lifted from their hearts. Tell me. Did we not love mankind when we admitted so humbly its impotence and lovingly lightened its burden . . . ? (40)

or by siding with the moral philosopher Berlin:

> . . . to manipulate men, to propel them toward goals which you—the social reformer [or psychiatrist]—see, but they may not, is to deny their human essence, to treat them as objects without wills of their own, and therefore to degrade them. That is why . . . to use [human beings] as means for my, not their own independently conceived ends, even if it is for their own benefit is, in effect, to treat them as sub-human, to behave as if their ends are less ultimate and sacred than my own (41).

Informed consent, like other concepts which convey an uncritical optimism about human capacities for making responsible choices and for being respectful of other persons' choices, is easily prone to corruption by an equally uncritical pessimism about human capacities to be choice-makers. Dostoyevsky and Berlin present these conflicting views about human capacities unswervingly and starkly. While both views express something profound about human nature and human aspirations which deserve serious consideration, it does not necessarily follow that one cannot adopt one rather than the other as a guiding principle.

In today's world, the Grand Inquisitor's view predominates and this choice has made informed consent the confusing doctrine it is. If one wishes to bow to his wisdom, let it be acknowledged and go on from there. It is far more respectful of ourselves and our patients to do so than to continue with the present charade of expressing a commitment to self-decision-making, which in fact does not exist. What parades today under informed consent victimizes both professionals and patients and this is particularly true in the practice of psychiatry which, after all, is supposed to be committed to helping patients assume greater responsibility for their conduct.

Berlin points us in a different direction. He wishes to take psychiatrists on an impossible mission, which, nevertheless, may be worth pursuing. To embark on it requires first of all a commitment to dialogue, to joint decision-making between psychiatrist and patient. Such a dialogue must be grounded in an awareness by both parties of their ignorance and limitations as well as of the uncertainties inherent in the state of the art.

Having spent many years reflecting on the problems which need to be resolved before meaningful dialogue can become possible, I have attempted in this essay to convey the complexity of the issues which need to be better understood. A ray of light, however, has begun to illuminate my work. Increasingly I am convinced that, though patients bring all kinds of incapacities to the dialogue, professionals have contributed their share to making collaboration in decision-making well-nigh impossible. If I am correct, we can begin by working on ourselves. How difficult an assignment this will turn out to be, remains to be seen.

Freud once wrote that the third great blow to man's narcissism was the realization that "the ego is not master in its house" (42). Underlying this observation is a question: To what extent can human beings engage in a dialogue with themselves in order to reconcile the rational and irrational residing within them? The command "physician heal thyself" takes on another meaning: to learn how to talk to ourselves before we commence to heal others. If we could learn that, then the impossible mission would become a possible one, for we may finally know how to talk *with* patients rather than *at* them.

To return once more to Dostoyevsky and Berlin. In attempting to follow Berlin's philosophy, we must also appreciate Dostoyevsky's observations—that patients may all too willingly "hand over . . . the gift of freedom," and that professionals may all too willingly "lighten [freedom's] burden." The idea of informed consent instructs us to resist both temptations.

REFERENCES

1. *Salgo v. Leland Stanford, Jr. University Board of Trustees,* 317 P.2d 170 (1957).
2. *Ibid.,* at 181.
3. Brief of American College of Surgeons as Amicus Curiae in Support of Defendant and Appellant Frank Gerbode (1959).
4. *Natanson v. Kline,* 350 P.2d 1093 (1960).
5. *Ibid.,* at 1104.
6. *Ibid.,* at 1106.
7. *Ibid.,* at 1103.
8. *Canterbury v. Spence,* 464 F.2d 772 (1972).
9. *Cobbs v. Grant,* 502 P.2d 1 (1972).
10. *Canterbury v. Spence,* at 790.
11. Louisiana Public Health and Safety Code 40:1299.40 (1975); Ohio Rev. Code Ann. §2317.54 (1976).
12. *McMullen v. Vaughan,* 227 S.E. 2d 440, 442 (1976).
13. *Scaria v. St. Paul Fire & Marine Ins. Co.,* 227 N.W.2d 647, 659 (1975).
14. Katz, J.: Informed Consent—A Fairy Tale? Law's Vision, 39 *Univ. of Pittsburgh Law Rev.* 137-74 (1977).
15. Oath of Hippocrates (5th century B.C.).
16. Hippocrates: *Decorum.* In *Hippocrates Vol. II.* (W. H. S. Jones translation). Cambridge: Harvard University Press, 1967, pp. 297-99.
17. Becker, H. S.: The Nature of a Profession. In: Henry, N. B., ed.: *The*

Sixty-First Yearbook of the National Society for the Study of Education. Chicago: The National Society for the Study of Education, 1962, p. 27.

18. American Medical Association: *Principles of Medical Ethics.* Chicago: American Medical Association (1969).
19. Parsons, T.: *The Social System.* Glencoe, Ill.: The Free Press (1951).
20. MacIntyre, A.: Patients as Agents. In: Spicker, S. F. and Engelhardt, H. T., eds.: *Philosophical Medical Ethics—Its Nature and Significance.* Boston: D. Reidel Publishing Co., 1977, pp. 197, 205.
21. Freud, S.: *New Introductory Lectures on Psycho-Analysis.* The Standard Edition of the Complete Psychological Works of Sigmund Freud, Vol. 17. London: The Hogarth Press, 1964.
22. Feinstein, A.: *Clinical Judgment.* Baltimore: The Williams and Wilkins Co., 1967, p. 23.
23. Marshall, E.: Psychotherapy Works, But for Whom? *Science,* 207:506-508, 1980.
24. *Rogers v. Okin,* 478 F. Supp. 1342 (1979).
25. Schaffer, P.: Court Rules that Mental Patients Have Right to Refuse Treatment, *Clinical Psychiatry News,* 8:1 (Jan. 1980).
26. *Rogers v. Okin,* at 1360.
27. *Ibid.* at 1361.
28. *Ibid.* at 1364.
29. *Ibid.* at 1367.
30. Burt, R.: *Taking Care of Strangers.* New York: The Free Press, 1979, p. 134.
31. *Rogers v. Okin,* at 1369.
32. Byerly, H.: Explaining and Exploiting Placebo Effects, *Perspectives of Biology and Medicine,* 423, 1976.
33. Houston, W. R.: The Doctor Himself as a Therapeutic Agent, *Annals of Internal Medicine,* 11:1415, 1938.
34. Hoffer, A.: A Theoretical Examination of Double-Blind Design, *Canadian Medical Association Journal,* 97:123, 1967.
35. Menninger, R.: Diagnosis of Culture and Social Institutions, *Bull. Menninger Clinic,* 40:531, 537, 1976.
36. Bird., B.: *Talking with Patients.* Philadelphia: J. B. Lippincott, 1973, pp. 14-15.
37. Freud, A.: The Doctor-Patient Relationship. In Katz. J.: *Experimentation with Human Beings.* New York: The Russell Sage Foundation, 1972, p. 637.
38. Mill, J. S.: *On Liberty.* Oxford: Basil Blackwell, 1946 ed., p. 68.
39. See Loewald, H.: On the Therapeutic Action of Psychoanalysis, *Int. J. of Psychoanalysis,* 41:16-33, 1960.
40. Dostoyevsky, F.: *The Brothers Karamazov.* Translated by D. Magarshack. Baltimore: Penguin Books, 1958, p. 301.
41. Berlin, I.: *Four Essays on Liberty.* Oxford: Clarendon Press, 1969.
42. Freud, S.: *A Difficulty in the Path of Psychoanalysis.* In Standard Edition of the Complete Psychological Works of Sigmund Freud, Vol. 17. London: The Hogarth Press, 1955, pp. 137, 143.

5

Tarasoff and the Duty to Warn Potential Victims

George E. Dix, J.D.

A recent newspaper item reported that a woman, Mary Cole, from Des Moines, Iowa had filed suit against her psychiatrist, seeking damages for harm caused when she killed her former husband in 1977. The suit alleged that the psychiatrist was negligent in a number of ways, including failure to examine Cole with sufficient care, failing to warn her former husband, police, or her present husband of the danger she posed, failing to hospitalize Cole, and failing in general to protect others from the danger created by Cole's illness. Cole had been convicted of murder for the killing of her ex-husband, the report noted (1).

As this lawsuit indicates, the dangerous proclivities of patients in therapy have become a matter of increasing discussion and litigation. Much of the discussion has been stimulated by a recent decision of the California Supreme Court, *Tarasoff v. Board of Regents* (2). This decision, which undoubtedly is being relied upon by Ms. Cole, indicated that psychiatrists and other therapists have a legal obligation to identify patients who pose a serious risk of physical harm to others and, under some circumstances at least, to contact those third persons directly and warn them of the risk.

The questions raised by *Tarasoff* are explored in this essay. First, the decision itself is examined. Attention is then turned to the ramifications of the decision and specifically the duties which a therapist may have to warn a potential victim. In the third section, the impact of *Tarasoff* upon the therapist's required disclosure for informed consent to therapy is scrutinized. The fourth section addresses the basic policy question that will inevitably be presented when courts in other jurisdictions are asked to follow *Tarasoff*—should *Tarasoff*-type liability exist? The concluding section considers the availability of reasonable alternatives to the so-called *Tarasoff* rule.

THE *TARASOFF* DECISION

In late 1969, Prosenjit Poddar was a patient of Dr. Lawrence Moore, a psychologist employed by a California university hospital mental health clinic. During therapy, Poddar made certain statements which caused Dr. Moore to believe that he posed a danger to a young woman named Tatiana Tarasoff. Dr. Moore consulted with a psychiatrist and then notified campus police that Poddar was dangerous and should be hospitalized. The police officers located Poddar, but, after discussing the matter with him, they decided that he was not dangerous and failed to take further action. Soon thereafter, the psychiatrist in charge of the clinic returned from an absence and was informed of these events. He directed that no further action be taken to hospitalize Poddar, asked the police to return Dr. Moore's written communication concerning Poddar, and ordered that all correspondence and records concerning the matter be destroyed. Poddar persuaded Tarasoff's brother to share an apartment near her residence, and, two months after the efforts by Dr. Moore to have him hospitalized, Poddar killed Tarasoff.

Tarasoff's parents brought suit against, among others, the therapists at the clinic. The trial court dismissed the suit before trial, concluding that even if the senior Tarasoffs established their allegations, the defendants were not liable. On appeal, the California Supreme Court reversed the decision (2). Because of a California statute, the court held, the therapists could not be held liable even if they were negligent in their efforts to secure Poddar's hospitalization. But, the court continued, therapists owe a duty to potential victims of dangerous patients, and this duty may be violated by failing to warn the victims of the danger posed by the patients. The plaintiffs were, therefore, entitled to an opportunity to prove that the defendant therapists were negligent in failing to warn Tarasoff. The case was remanded with directions to the trial judge to permit it to go to trial.

The procedural posture of the case is important because it makes clear the limited nature of the holding. The California Supreme Court did not hold that any of the defendants were in fact negligent in failing to warn the potential victim. It merely held that it was conceivable in law that failing to warn a potential victim could constitute actionable negligence, and that the plaintiffs were entitled to an opportunity to establish that, on the facts of the case, the defendants' failure to warn Tarasoff was negligence. After the decision of the state's highest court, the case was settled for an undisclosed amount. Consequently, the question of whether any of the therapists were, in fact, negligent was never litigated.

The decision does, however, establish two significant propositions as a matter of California law. First, it makes clear that therapists owe a duty of care not only to their patients but also to persons who might be harmed by these patients. Psychiatrists have traditionally owed their patients a duty of reasonable care, and if, as a result of a therapist's negligence, a patient harmed another person and was consequently harmed himself, the therapist was liable to the patient for the damage caused. In this sense, Ms. Cole's lawsuit described above—unlike the senior Tarasoffs' litigation—is based upon relatively traditional theories of liability.

The second proposition which the decision establishes is that a therapist's duty to third persons can be breached by—among other things—a failure to warn a potential victim. To put the matter negatively, the court rejected the proposition that under no possible circumstances could a failure to warn a potential victim constitute a violation of the therapist's duty to the potential victim. There *may* be some situations, the court speculated, in which a therapist would be liable for failing to warn the victim. Insofar as Ms. Cole's lawsuit relies upon the defendant-therapist's failure to warn her former husband as the basis for liability, it is based upon one of the relatively novel aspects of the *Tarasoff* holding.

Neither of these propositions are binding in any other jurisdiction as a result of the decision. The California Supreme Court is, however, well-regarded among American courts, and it is reasonable to expect the *Tarasoff* decision to be an influential consideration for other courts that might be called upon to address the same or similar issues in the future. To some extent, California can be regarded as an experiment in practice under a duty to warn. A study by Wise of the effects of *Tarasoff* in California provides some assistance in determining the effects of the duty imposed by that decision; these will be discussed in more detail later (3). It is useful to note at this point, however, the high interest in and relevance of the decision. Wise reports that one year after the California Supreme Court's decision, 96% of the psychiatrists surveyed had heard of the decision and 80% reported seeing at least one potentially dangerous patient each year.

Though the desirability or acceptability of the *Tarasoff* result will be explored later in this paper, two matters are of such special importance to this question that they will be examined separately in the next two sections. The first is the specific effect of *Tarasoff*: When, under that decision, does a therapist violate his/her legal obligation to potential victims and become liable for any harm caused? The second concerns the effect of possible disclosure upon the therapist-patient relationship: When, under *Tarasoff*, must a therapist tell a potential or actual patient that the therapist may be required to warn persons whom he/she believes to be placed at risk by the patient's condition?

THE THERAPIST'S OBLIGATION
UNDER *TARASOFF*

Quite obviously, a major consideration in evaluating the desirability of *Tarasoff*-like liability is the obligation it imposes upon a therapist. Unfortunately, this is impossible to discuss with specificity. Because of the procedural posture of the case, the decision of the California Supreme Court offers little guidance on even the question of whether, given the apparent facts of that case, the defendant-therapists' actions in general—and their failure to warn Tarasoff in particular—constituted actionable negligence. The court's language, however, makes clear that it regards the issue as calling for the application of the general malpractice standard:

> [O]nce a therapist does in fact determine, or under applicable professional standards reasonably should have determined, that a patient poses a serious danger of violence to others, he bears a duty to exercise reasonable care to protect the foreseeable victim of that danger. While the discharge of this duty of due care will necessarily vary with the facts of each case, in each instance the adequacy of the therapist's conduct must be measured against the traditional negligence standard of reasonable care under the circumstances (2, p. 345).

This statement of the *Tarasoff* court's holding makes two things clear. First, no duty to act arises until the therapist determines a patient presents a serious danger of violence or until circumstances are such that a reasonable professional would make such a determination. Second, once a duty arises, it can be discharged in several ways, only one of which need involve warning the potential victim (4). While *Tarasoff* recognizes the possibility that the duty may be breached by failing to warn the victim, it clearly does not hold that the only way to comply with the duty is to warn the potential victim. In a sense, then, the title of this essay is misleading. Even under *Tarasoff* there is nothing that can properly be called a "duty to warn;" the relevant duty is to exercise reasonable care to preserve the safety of potential victims, and warning the victim is only one of several ways that a therapist can perform this duty. Ms. Cole's lawsuit apparently takes this into account and does not rely exclusively upon the defendant-therapist's failure to warn her now deceased former husband of the danger posed by Ms. Cole. Rather, the allegation appears to be that the therapist was negligent in failing to act in any acceptable way to preserve the safety of her former husband; she alleges that the defendant did not warn him, notify police, hospitalize her, or in any other fashion act to safeguard her potential victim.

In regard to making the determination of dangerousness and deciding how to act upon it, the therapist is not held to accuracy. It is only necessary that the therapist's actions come within the range of professional acceptability. As the court stated:

> Within the broad range of reasonable practice and treatment in which professional opinion and judgment may differ, the therapist is free to exercise his or her own best judgment without liability; proof, aided by hindsight, that he or she judged wrongly is insufficient to establish negligence (2, p. 345).

These statements are obviously quite general. Can anything more specific be said? Since there is no appellate case law and no reported trial court experience dealing with application of *Tarasoff*, further discussion will necessarily be highly speculative. The most that can be done is the identification of factors which are potentially relevant to the issues. In doing this, however, it is necessary to keep in mind that there are two distinct issues posed by *Tarasoff*, or, to put the matter another way, under *Tarasoff*, a therapist has two distinct duties. First, the therapist has a duty to exercise reasonable care in identifying patients who pose a danger to third persons. Second, the therapist has a duty, once a dangerous patient has been—or should have been—identified, to take reasonable precautions to protect the potential victim. A breach of duty, i.e., a failure to exercise reasonable care in identifying a dangerous patient, or a failure to take reasonable care in protecting a potential victim, can give rise to liability, if it results in harm to the victim.

Whether either duty has been violated in a particular case will be determined by applying a standard of professional competence. In regard to the first matter, then, the issue will be whether a therapist who did not identify a patient as dangerous failed to exercise the care and skill generally exercised by mental health professionals in identifying dangerous patients. In regard to the second matter, the issue is whether, in deciding how to respond to the situation presented when a dangerous patient has been (or should have been) identified, the therapist exercised the care and skill generally brought to bear on such situations by mental health professionals.

What follows is an effort to identify the wide variety of considerations relevant to determining the reasonableness of a therapist's behavior in a *Tarasoff*-like situation. All bear upon how a reasonable mental health professional will respond to such situations. They are all also factors that courts are likely to find relevant in deciding whether a mental health professional's response (or nonresponse) gives rise to liability under *Tarasoff*. It is important to note that some bear upon the identification of a patient as "dangerous," some are relevant to the therapist's response to a patient identified as dangerous, and some apply to both of those matters.

1) *Therapist's Contribution to Risk.* If the therapist has contributed to the risk involved, this fact will increase the therapist's responsibility, especially if the therapist's contribution to the risk is the result of what is itself a breach of professional standards. Conceivably, both *Tarasoff* duties might be affected by this. If the therapist has in some way increased the danger which the patient poses to others, the therapist will be required to exercise greater care in judging the patient's dangerousness than would otherwise be the case. Moreover, the therapist will be held to a somewhat higher standard of care in deciding how to act upon that risk once it is identified. In *Tarasoff*, for example, it is possible that the supervising psychiatrist countermanded the initial efforts to hospitalize Poddar without adequate consultation with those staff persons familiar with the case and without an adequate personal

evaluation of Poddar. If this was the case, the supervising psychiatrist's actions contributed to the risk to the victim and suggest that the therapist was professionally negligent both in failing to identify Poddar as dangerous to Tarasoff and in failing to warn Tarasoff concerning this danger.

2) *Kind of Harm Anticipated.* Obviously, the more severe the harm anticipated, the more likely the patient is to be "dangerous" and the more likely some preventive action—perhaps, including a warning—is indicated. It is equally obvious that there will often be difficulty in predicting the specific injury likely to occur to the victim. However, in situations in which the therapist has reason to fear that the patient will seek to inflict a gunshot wound on the victim, a warning is more strongly indicated than when the therapist has reason to believe that the patient will only slap the victim.

3) *Likelihood of Harm.* The more likely it appears to be that the patient will cause the harm the more important identification of the patient as dangerous and protective action become. This, of course, presents the problem of predicting in terms of comparative likelihoods. The present paper is not the place to develop the factors relevant to the difficult or perhaps impossible task of evaluating the likelihood of assaultive behavior. It is virtually certain, however, that courts will look to such factors as the extent to which the patient has engaged in similar action in the past, any threats made by the patient (and the specificity of these threats), any indication to the therapist that the patient has made specific plans for the assault, and similar matters.

4) *Specificity of Danger Posed.* A major factor in determining the professionally indicated response to a patient identified as dangerous is likely to be the extent to which the danger perceived by the therapist is focused upon one or a small number of victims. The more focused the danger, the more a warning is indicated. In *Tarasoff*, for example, it was clear that the major danger posed by Poddar was to a single person, readily identifiable. If the

defendant-therapists had instead perceived a significant danger that Poddar would respond violently to some innocuous aspect of interaction with others, a warning would have been far less indicated. In part, this is because the more diffuse the danger, the less feasible (or more burdensome) warning becomes. In addition, however, the more subjects that must be warned, the more significant the breach of confidentiality and therefore the more "costly" the warning. Of course, if a therapist perceives a significant danger of severe harm to a diffuse group of victims but no duty to warn exists, the therapist's duty may well be to take other preventive action, such as beginning hospitalization proceedings or notifying law enforcement authorities.

5) *Duration of Risk.* The longer the duration of the risk which the therapist perceives—or should perceive—the patient as presenting, the more important it is to identify the patient as dangerous. Thus, no duty to take preventive action may arise when the risk is a short-term one, occasioned by some fleeting aspect of the patient's life. On the other hand, if circumstances are such that the same risk will exist for a prolonged period, preventive action may be necessary.

6) *Consent of the Patient.* If a dangerous patient has consented to the therapist's warning the potential victim, this may suggest that the appropriate professional response is such a warning. Cases reported by Roth and Meisel indicate that, in a substantial number of cases, the therapist can obtain the patient's consent to contact a potential victim (5).

At first glance, the consent of the patient to the breach of confidentiality would seem to resolve the matter completely. This, however, is an oversimplification. Depending upon the situation, reliance upon consent raises the danger that the consent will subsequently be found legally ineffective. Especially if obtained during the course of therapy, consent elicited by the therapist's persuasion may be regarded as involuntary and thus of no legal effect. The therapist must also, of course, be sensitive to the ethical problem of the nature of persuasion that can and should be utilized to secure a consent for what might be regarded as serving only the self-interest of the therapist in avoiding liability. In addition, the warning or any other direct contact between the therapist and the potential victim may signicantly interfere with the therapeutic relationship and hence with the effectiveness of therapy (6). It seems clear that the therapist's duty to the patient requires that the therapist not seek the patient's consent to warn a potential victim unless the therapist, after full consideration, has made a reasonable determination that the potential impact of the warning on the therapy is an acceptable price to pay.

7) *Harm to Danger-reducing Therapeutic Relationship.* If the therapist perceives that s/he still has a meaningful relationship with a patient identified by the therapist as dangerous, that continued therapy would reduce the danger posed by the patient, and that giving a warning would harm or destroy that relationship, a warning may not be necessary or appropriate. In evaluating this consideration, however, the therapist must be careful not to assume uncritically that warning will result in destruction of the therapeutic relationship. The therapist must creatively consider the possibility that the warning process might be used to therapeutic benefit.

Stone emphasizes the potential damage a warning may do to therapy. He suggests that patients who pose danger will often be persons experiencing passion or paranoia regarding a person of intense significance to them. In such situations, he continues, the therapist must maintain an attitude of respect for and acceptance of the patient's feelings while discouraging violent action on them. The therapist's delicate position, he then concludes, will be especially endangered if the therapist gives the patient the impression that a significant relationship exists between the object of the patient's passions and the therapist (6). A warning, of course, might well create such an impression and thus bode ill for the future of the therapeutic relationship. Wexler, however, suggests that there may be significant therapeutic value in placing increased emphasis upon the role of the potential victim and in seeking out acceptable ways of obtaining information from potential victims. Thus, the therapist might seek and secure the patient's consent to contact the potential victim and through this contact might obtain information of significant value to the therapy (7). It is not unreasonable to consider the possibility of involving the potential victim in the therapy. In any case, while Stone's cautions are certainly not to be ignored, the therapist must also consider the possibility that contact with the potential victim, if skillfully managed, may in fact enhance the effectiveness of the therapy.

8) *Patient-Victim Relationship.* The relationship between the patient and the possible victim is relevant to both responsibilities of the therapist. If the relationship between the patient and a possible victim is a close one, this suggests that the patient should be identified as dangerous, since the relationship may provide opportunities for the patient to harm the victim. In addition, such a relationship may indicate that a warning rather than some other response is appropriate once the patient has been identified as dangerous. If the warning is given to one with whom the defendant has a close relationship, this may minimize the seriousness of the breach of confidentiality. The patient may perceive the intrusiveness of disclosure to such a person as relatively minimal and such a person might reasonably be expected to avoid further dissemination of the confidential information contained in the warning.

9) *Value of Warning to Victim.* In deciding how to respond to a patient identified as dangerous, the therapist must assess the apparent value that a warning will have to the victim. From the information available to the therapist, is the victim likely to respond to the warning by taking action that will reduce the risk? If the victim is already aware that the patient has expressed violent thoughts or intentions concerning him/her, this may indicate that a warning is not appropriate. On the other hand, the therapist must not overlook the possibility that a potential victim, who is aware of threats or similar indications of danger, may, if warned by a therapist, be caused to take these indications more seriously and perhaps be stirred to significant pro-

tective action. If, of course, the potential victim appears to have no realization that the patient poses a threat to him/her, this indicates that a warning is required.

10) *Adverse Impact Upon Potential Victim.* In deciding how to respond to a dangerous patient, a therapist must also consider the possibility that a warning will have an adverse impact upon the potential victim and even, indirectly, upon the patient. Griffith and Griffith emphasize that a warning of the sort suggested in *Tarasoff* might cause fear and anxiety in the potential victim and raise the possibility that the therapist might conceivably be liable for negligently causing mental distress by improperly warning a potential victim (8). Moreover, they suggest that a warning may stimulate a potential victim into becoming the aggressor, thereby causing a violent confrontation between the patient and the potential victim in which the potential victim, the patient, or both, may be injured. In deciding whether to warn, a therapist must, of course, consider this possible adverse side effect as one factor bearing upon whether a warning is indicated.

11) *Available Alternatives to Warning.* In deciding upon a course of action, once a patient has been identified as dangerous, a therapist must consider possible alternatives to warning the victim, their likely effectiveness, and their cost in all relevant terms. The major alternatives, of course, are hospitalization proceedings and notice to law enforcement authorities. The therapist must consider such matters as his/her ability to secure hospitalization, the likelihood that such action will reduce the danger posed to the potential victim, and costs such as the impact of such action upon the therapist's relationship with the patient. In *Tarasoff*, for example, at least some of the defendants had found both hospitalization and notice to law enforcement authorities to be unavailable or at least of no apparent value, given local laws and attitudes. Thus, the possible absence of alternatives may have indicated that the duty owed to the potential victim could be respected only by a warning.

In some cases, acceptable alternatives that do not require going beyond the therapeutic relationship may be presented. Roth and

Meisel, for example, suggest that, in some situations, requiring the patient to rid himself of dangerous weapons may be enough (5). (The therapist would be well advised, of course, to obtain some reasonable assurance that a patient has complied with such a request or demand.) In some cases, a therapist might reasonably conclude that continued therapy alone, or with some modification of approach, holds sufficient promise of eliminating the danger to make it a viable alternative to warning the potential victim.

12) *Patient's Acceptance of Limits of Confidentiality.* Many of the possible responses to a dangerous patient involve breaches of confidentiality. To the extent that the patient has been informed that confidentiality is not absolute and has continued with therapy understanding this, responses that breach confidentiality are acceptable, if necessary. Conversely, if no such understanding exists, these alternatives are less acceptable ones. Of course, the therapist's choice from among the alternatives that involve breach of confidentiality may be affected by the understanding of the patient. Warning a potential victim, for example, is acceptable if the patient was specifically told such a warning might be regarded by the therapist as necessary. If the patient was only told in a general way that in extreme situations the therapist might be required to breach confidentiality, a warning would be less appropriate.

In deciding what significance to give the patient's apparent acceptance of limits on confidentiality, the therapist must consider the extent to which the patient's continued disclosure of confidences in therapy constitutes a voluntary and understanding acceptance of the risk of disclosure. When the patient apparently understands the possibility of disclosure and when his decision to continue does not seem closely related to his psychopathology, the therapist can give more weight to the patient's acceptance.

A word of caution: I do not suggest that a failure to inform the patient that a potential victim-warning may be necessary will mean that a warning is never acceptable. (This aspect is discussed in more detail in the next section.) It is, however, important to note that the dangerous patient's awareness and acceptance of possible exceptions to absolute confidentiality are factors which the therapist must take into account in deciding how to respond.

13) *Impact of Alternatives Upon Patient's General Well-Being.* In deciding how to respond to a patient identified as dangerous, a therapist is entitled to consider the impact of possible responses upon the patient's general well-being. Civil commitment has obvious stigma effects. Perhaps most important, if the therapist reasonably believes that warning the potential victim will destroy the possibility of continued therapy and that continued therapy will enable the patient to live a more satisfactory life, the therapist may consider this as indicating that such a warning is not an appropriate response. This consideration differs from number 7 above in that it does not bear upon the likelihood of the various alternatives reducing the risk to the victim. While *Tarasoff* requires the therapist to give significant weight to the interest of potential victims, it does not mandate that the therapist ignore what appear to be the patient's own best interests.

14) *Results of Consultations with Others.* One result of *Tarasoff* and similar cases may be to encourage therapists who are confronted with potentially dangerous patients to consult with others. Wise's survey of California therapists disclosed that following *Tarasoff* there was some increase in therapists' consultation with other professionals regarding potentially dangerous patients (3). If this is done, the results of those consultations are relevant to whether the therapist is required to regard the patient as dangerous and, if so, what response is indicated. Most consultations are likely to be with other mental health professionals; if these other professionals indicate that in their judgment the danger is less than the therapist feared, or that the results of disclosure would be more harmful than the therapist anticipated, this indicates that a warning may be less necessary. Consultation may also, of course, be with an attorney. "Ignorance of the law is no excuse," and it seems clear that being advised by a lawyer that no duty to act exists (on specific facts) does not mean that no duty in fact exists. Yet if a therapist in good faith seeks

legal advice and is told that no legal duty to act exists, this again is a factor to be considered in determining whether the therapist's failure to take further precautions was unreasonable.

15) *Impact of Disclosure Upon Other Patients.* Obviously, the major considerations bearing upon the appropriate response to a dangerous patient are those presented by the specific situation before the therapist. To some extent, however, a reasonable therapist must consider the long-range impact of the various alternatives. Thus, a therapist may reasonably believe that giving a warning in a particular case will result in the breach of confidentiality becoming generally known, and that this will result in other patients being less willing to enter into therapeutic relationships. If a therapist believes that a warning will endanger his/her therapeutic relationships, a warning may not be the most appropriate course of action. Conversely, if it reasonably appears that the warning could be given without endangering other patients' therapeutic relationships, this suggests that a warning may be appropriate.

16) *General and Local Practice.* The therapist may, of course, properly consider local and more general practice both in deciding whether a patient is dangerous and in deciding how to respond to a dangerous patient. If, for example, such practice is to give warnings in situations that appear similar, this suggests that a warning is required.

Some argue that, at least in the absence of a *Tarasoff*-like decision, therapists uniformly respect confidentiality (at least in regard to potential victims), and that, therefore, there are no professional standards regarding when to warn. There are indications, however, that this is simply not so. Slovenko, minimizing the effects of *Tarasoff*, states that "it has long been the general practice" to discretely warn "appropriate" persons in some situations where a patient presents a threat (9). Wise found that, even before *Tarasoff*, therapists in California warned potential victims. Nevertheless, she found grounds for concluding that the *Tarasoff* decision did have an impact upon warning practices. Some—but "only very tenuous"—evidence suggested that the frequency of warnings increased in the year following *Tarasoff*. More substantial evidence indicated a shift in the persons warned. After *Tarasoff*, according to the respondents, therapists were more likely than before to warn the potential victim rather than the patient's family or law enforcement authorities (3). It seems quite likely that, despite the likelihood that a *Tarasoff*-like decision would change therapists' warning practices to some extent, a case can be made for the proposition that there are informal standards, based on present practice, for determining when a potential victim should be warned.

If, however, local practice were indeed never to communicate risks to potential victims, this would appear a relevant consideration suggesting that no duty existed. But this must be considered with caution. The significance of decisions such as *Tarasoff* may be—if practice is never or seldom to warn potential victims—to indicate that for legal purposes existing general practice is itself unreasonable and therefore cannot be relied upon. In other words, the decision of the court may be a declaration that professional standards cannot be judged solely by existing practice and that some limited aspects of existing practice may no longer be acceptable. Nevertheless, existing practice—especially in the particular locality—is relevant and may be considered, although therapists should be cautious before giving it controlling significance.

17) *Presumption Favoring Confidentiality*. In doubtful cases, a therapist may have an ethical duty to preserve confidentiality. Moreover, that ethical responsibility may well have legal significance. The annotations to the *Principles of Medical Ethics*, when dealing with the therapist's responses to court-ordered disclosure, state: "When the psychiatrist is in doubt, the right of the patient to confidentiality, and, by extension, to unimpaired treatment, should be given priority" (10). By analogy, if a therapist is in doubt as to how to respond to the situation presented by a dangerous patient, it is reasonable to look favorably upon those options that involve no or little infringement upon confidentiality. In some situations, this may mean that warnings are properly

regarded as the least attractive alternative. The therapist must, however, realistically consider the infringement upon confidentiality involved in the alternatives. It is not beyond the realm of possibility, for example, for notice to law enforcement authorities to constitute a greater breach of confidentiality than a discreetly-made warning to a potential victim. This will certainly not in itself be of controlling legal significance, but a reasonable therapist can properly give some weight to an ethical presumption in favor of nondisclosure.

As was stressed above, these are all simply considerations that are likely to be found relevant to the two *Tarasoff* issues. It is unlikely that any one of them will be conclusive in any situation. The question will be whether, taking into account all of these considerations, the therapist's failure to take further or different precautions against harm to the victim was beyond the broad range of reasonable mental health practice.

INFORMED CONSENT TO THERAPY
UNDER *TARASOFF*

If a duty to warn potential victims exists, when, if ever, must therapists inform patients that they may be compelled to breach confidentiality by making such a warning? The question is important for several reasons. A psychiatrist who undertakes to give a required warning might conceivably become liable for a breach of confidentiality, if the patient has been encouraged to make disclosures without advance notice that the therapist may reveal those disclosures. In addition, the adverse impact that a duty to warn may have upon therapy may depend upon the extent of a patient-warning required. While it is possible that the mere existence of a duty to warn potential victims may have an adverse impact upon the therapist-patient relationship, the impact seems almost certain to be greater if therapists begin the relationship by stressing this exception to confidentiality.

Amazingly little consideration has been given to this point. Fleming and Maximov, whose work was apparently quite influential in the California Supreme Court *Tarasoff* decision, argue that therapy should be undertaken only after the therapist has specifically informed the patient of the possible duty to warn potential victims and thereafter secured the patient's now *informed* consent to therapy and attendant disclosures (11). Stone uncritically assumes that Fleming and Maximov are correct and that a duty to make such disclosure—apparently in all cases —would exist (6). Griffith and Griffith note that a therapist "might" have to warn the patient, but they undertake no discussion of the matter (8). There has apparently been little or no critical consideration of the possibility that these discussions may have been oversimplistic.

The reason for this situation may be the abysmal state of the law defining what is necessary for informed consent to psychiatric treatment. In general, courts state that physicians need not disclose all risks of treatment but only those risks disclosed by physicians within the community in their customary practice (12, 13). Under *Tarasoff*, whether therapists must disclose the possibility of warning potential victims depends in part upon whether therapists, in general, disclose this risk and upon the extent to which they disclose similar limitations upon confidentiality. Under the so-called "therapeutic privilege," a physician may withhold information from a patient, if the physician has reason to believe that disclosure of the information might cause the patient to forego the treatment or might increase the risk to the patient (12). Whether a therapist is entitled to invoke the therapeutic privilege as a basis for failing to disclose his/her obligation to warn potential victims will also depend in part upon current professional standards. Would a reasonable therapist, on the facts given, regard disclosure of the information as involving sufficient risk of harm to the patient as to justify nondisclosure? Obviously, prevailing disclosure practice is of paramount importance.

It is by no means clear that present practice involves routine disclosure of the duty to warn potential victims. In part, of course, this may be because most therapists have assumed that the duty does not exist—although the evidence cited above indicates that therapists have followed an ethical requirement of warning victims. Perhaps more helpful would be an inquiry into whether therapists generally warn patients about other limits on confidentiality that clearly exist in the psychiatric context; i.e., the therapist's duty to seek involuntary commitment of the patient (and in the process breach confidentiality if that becomes necessary) and to notify law enforcement officers or other authorities if those actions become necessary to protect others. If these exceptions to confidentiality are not routinely explained to patients, it is not apparent why a "new" exception covering warnings of potential victims need be explained. Moreover, if therapists believe that disclosure of this new risk would impede effective treatment, the therapeutic privilege may permit them to avoid explaining the duty to warn, especially on the facts of particular cases.

Wise's study is relevant. Her respondents indicated that their patients perceived confidentiality as being absolute even though the therapists recognized that it was not. Nevertheless, only 11% of the therapists reported that they "almost always" discussed confidentiality with patients. Seventy percent indicated that they discussed it "sometimes," meaning "if it comes up in therapy" (3). The implication is that under pre-*Tarasoff* California practice, therapists did not routinely undertake discussion of confidentiality with their patients and certainly did not specifically inform them of the then-existing limitations upon confidentiality. However, 20% of the respondents reported that following *Tarasoff* they more frequently discussed confidentiality with their patients; the reasons for this were not investigated in her study.

The only fair conclusion, then, is that it is unclear to what extent a duty to warn potential victims would also impose a duty upon therapists to warn all patients at the beginning of therapy concerning this possibility. An argument can be made that patients are ethically and perhaps legally entitled to this information, but there is a high likelihood that courts would, at least in the absence of aggravated circumstances, accept the explanation that a therapist wanted to avoid discouraging the patient from undergoing treatment or wanted to prevent the development of an attitude which would render treatment less effective. Until there are further developments, it is improper to assume that full disclosure is routinely required.

Roth and Meisel agree that not every patient accepted for therapy needs to be told of the *Tarasoff* exception to confidentiality, if it is applicable. They suggest, however, that if, during the course of therapy, facts develop which indicate to the therapist that the case may be one of the "infrequent" ones in which a duty to warn may develop, the therapist should explain to the patient the possibility that the therapist might be obligated to act (5). This approach has the obvious advantage of making the warning unnecessary in most cases and thus avoiding the harm that might flow from routine warnings to patients at the beginning of therapy. On the other hand, if Stone is correct, this approach may be problematic because it would mean interfering with the therapeutic relationship when it is most vulnerable. The patient would be informed of the possibility of contact between the therapist and the object of his hostile feelings at a time when his emotions may be at highest peak. This would seem to pose maximum danger to the therapeutic relationship.

Moreover, it is not clear what legal or ethical significance such a warning would have with respect to disclosures that involve confidential communications made by the patient *before* the warning. Certainly, the patient cannot be said to have in any meaningful way "consented" to disclosure at the therapist's option by having shared the earlier confidences. Perhaps Roth and Meisel are suggesting that the therapist give the patient the following option: "I believe that if you continue in therapy with me, I may have an obligation to breach confidentiality by warning X that you pose a danger to him. I am willing to continue your therapy, but only if you agree to authorize me to warn X if I decide this is appropriate. If you are unwilling to grant me this authority, I can no longer continue to treat you." If this is the purpose, it would seem necessary that the matter be put directly to the patient in these terms. Merely informing the patient of the therapist's possible duty to warn would be inadequate, given the danger that the patient may not fully understand the options available to him or her. Of course, this approach does not address the problem posed if a therapist receives sufficient information creating the duty to warn before an opportunity arises to inform the patient of this exception to confidentiality. In such situations, the therapist's duty may require a warning even if the patient opts to terminate therapy rather than authorize the therapist to warn the potential victim.

SHOULD *TARASOFF*-TYPE LIABILITY EXIST?

Even under *Tarasoff*, as I have indicated, there is no legal obligation that can accurately be called a "duty to warn." Widespread formulation of the basic issue in terms of the propriety of a duty to warn justifies continued use of that phraseology, but it is important to keep in mind that the questions are really different and more complex. They are:

1) Should the law permit a person injured by a patient to sue the patient's therapist on the grounds that the therapist negligently failed to recognize the risk posed by the patient?
2) Should the law permit therapists to be found negligent for failing to take adequate steps to protect potential victims from patients identified as dangerous and, specifically, for failing to warn potential victims if that can be shown on the facts of the particular case to have been the only professionally reasonable response?

The basic arguments in favor of imposing a duty to warn upon therapists can be quite simply stated. Therapists are in a unique position because they can foresee extremely dangerous conduct on the part of their patients. Consequently, the law should provide an incentive for them to anticipate such conduct, and, when it is anticipated, to take reasonable steps to prevent it. If therapists fail to exercise reasonable care to prevent assaultive acts by their patients, they should bear at least part of the financial responsibility for the patients' conduct. Imposing a duty to warn potential victims of dangerous patients if appropriate creates such an incentive and constitutes a reasonable method of imposing financial liability upon those therapists who fail to exercise reasonable care. The imposition of this burden is not unreasonable, since it amounts to no more than requiring that therapists conform to standards of care already followed by the majority of competent therapists.

The arguments against imposing such a duty are somewhat more complex. First, it can be argued that therapists have insufficient skill in predicting dangerous behavior—by their patients or others—to justify singling them out for imposing a duty to protect potential victims. This has been the position of the American Psychiatric Association in the *Tarasoff* litigation, and it is argued forcefully by Stone (6). In another context, Stone reviews the literature and concludes that mental health professionals have not been demonstrated to have any greater ability than to identify a high risk group of persons, less than half of whom would—in the absence of intervention—commit a dangerous act (14). A follow-up study found that, of persons "diagnosed" dangerous by mental health clinicians but nevertheless released to the community by courts, only 35% were found to have committed a serious assaultive crime during the five-year follow-up period (15). Monahan (16), after reviewing the research available, states that:

> The conclusion to emerge most strikingly from these studies is the great degree to which violence is overpredicted. Of those predicted to be dangerous, between 54 and 99 percent are false positives—people who will not, in fact, be found to have committed a dangerous act (p. 250).

According to this argument, since therapists who undertake to predict dangerous behavior are more often wrong than right, there is no justification for holding them liable for failing to predict or for failing to act upon an impression they may form concerning their patients.

Several responses to this argument are possible. One is an almost vindictive one that might be called the "just desserts" argument. Mental health professionals have, for years, been willing to offer predictions of dangerousness when called upon in other legal contexts, such as civil commitment proceedings and criminal sentencing processes. Consequently, they should not be allowed to deny their predictive abilities in this context. *Tarasoff*-type liability, in other words, is "just desserts" for therapists who have been assuming responsibility, perhaps improperly, for predicting behavior in other contexts. A New Jersey court (17), explaining its decision to follow *Tarasoff*, was clearly influenced by this sort of consideration:

> Unless therapists clearly state when called upon to treat patients or to testify that they have no ability to predict or even determine whether their treatment will be efficacious or may even be necessary with any degree of certainty, there is no basis for a legal conclusion negating any and all duty [to predict behavior] with respect to a particular class of professionals (p. 508).

Of course, this pronouncement fails to meet the issue. If in fact clinical predictive ability is nonexistent, the appropriate remedy is not that of relying upon it in imposing tort liability upon therapists and continuing to rely upon it in hospitalization and criminal proceedings. The appropriate action is to avoid imposition of a tort duty and to reconsider the propriety of continued reliance upon predictive ability in other contexts.

Another possible response is that, despite the absence of empirical evidence, clinical predictions are at least sufficiently accurate to justify reliance upon them in this context as well as in civil commitment proceedings and criminal litigation. This position has been urged by Holbrook, who finds "historical data" (apparently the traditional acceptance of and reliance upon clinical testimony in litigation) which cannot be statistically validated as sufficiently establishing the accuracy of clinical predictions. He argues:

> [W]e are already making these judgments [concerning dangerousness] in a much larger area than the "duty to warn" would provide for. We cannot now abdicate responsibility in these areas because of institutional psychiatry taking what appears to be a strong position against the "duty to warn" proposition. This is not going to make our respon-

sibility as behavioral science practitioners go away (18, p. 705).

Moreover, there is reason to doubt that the evidence of psychiatric inability to predict dangerousness applies to all situations in which dangerousness is at issue. The studies to date have been almost exclusively concerned with long-term predictions concerning persons who have engaged in criminal activity. Yet the therapist upon whom the burden of a *Tarasoff*-like duty would fall is most likely to be confronted with the problem in a far different context, where the concern is with the short-term behavior of a person without an extensive criminal history. Furthermore, the studies have evaluated efforts by institutional staff to predict the behavior of institutionalized subjects, after those subjects had returned to the community. Monahan argues that such efforts are quite likely to be among the least successful attempts at prediction (19). The task that *Tarasoff* would require of mental health professionals is more akin to that presented when a prospective patient is evaluated for purposes of determining whether short-term emergency hospitalization is warranted. Monahan finds impressive reasons for concluding that the circumstances presented by the evaluation of a person for purposes of determining the short-term risk that he/she poses to others while in the community "may be exempt from the systematic inaccuracy found in the current [prediction] research." Consequently, he concludes, there are simply no data on the accuracy of such evaluations (19). In other words, while we do not know how accurate mental health professionals are in predicting assaultiveness in *Tarasoff*-like situations, there is reason to believe that it is a mistake to completely accept the available evidence as indicating no ability to predict.

A second argument against the duty to warn is that it poses an impossible burden on therapists. Reliance upon purportedly existing professional standards, Stone argues, is impossible, because the lack of an ability to predict dangerous behavior means there is no present standard of professional care (6). In addition, the duty to warn leaves the precise requirements imposed upon therapists unclear. Holbrook, for example, wonders whether a therapist who warns a potential victim also has a duty to advise that person as to how the threat might best be met (18). It is unclear whether a single warning will suffice and, if not, when additional warnings need to be given. Uncertainty exists as to what, if any, information the therapist must provide to the potential victim in addition to the existence of the therapist's concern. Griffith and Griffith, concerned with the danger that the potential victim might respond to the warning by attacking the patient, suggest the possibility that the therapist might have to warn the patient that the potential victim has been warned (18). Since existing professional standards and practices provide no basis for judging when and how a reasonable therapist would warn a potential victim, particular therapists should never be required to defend their failures to warn on the basis that they failed to conform to professional standards.

There are possible responses to this argument. If in fact there are no existing professional standards, this circumstance should become clear in litigation. In the event that this is established, litigation should cease, because lawyers would become aware of the impossibility of establishing the standard that defendants have arguably breached. More likely, however, litigation will show substantial disagreement concerning the methods of prediction but will also make clear that a significant number of mental health professionals do undertake to predict dangerous conduct according to a rather wide range of criteria. The resulting discussion of whether predictions should be made and, if so, how they should be accomplished cannot help but benefit both the profession and society by encouraging discussion about this important issue. In regard to the uncertainty concerning the scope of therapists' obligation under the duty, the problem can be regarded as at most a transitory one. Litigation under the new duty will result in these issues being clarified. The transitional uncertainty is unfortunate, but it is an inevitable result of the development of new legal doctrines.

A third argument against the duty to warn is related to the second. Given the absence of professional standards dealing with prediction of dangerous behavior and appropriate responses to a dangerous patient, courts will be unable to administer the duty to warn in a consistent and fair way. As a result, liability will be imposed inconsistently and arbitrarily. In other words, since courts cannot enforce the duty fairly, they should not enforce it at all.

In response, it can be argued that professional standards concerning identification of and responses to dangerous patients either exist at present or will develop from the concern and discussion likely to be engendered by the duty to warn. If reasonably fair application of the duty cannot be assured, then the duty can be abandoned; but, at present, there is no reason to abandon attempts at even-handed application of the duty.

The final argument against imposition of a duty to warn is that, whatever may be the advantages that flow from the duty, there are far greater costs or disadvantages. One cost is the infringement upon the privacy of the patient. Another, discussed above, is the impact upon the potential victims: The warning may cause them significant discomfort and could conceivably stimulate assaultive actions that would not otherwise take place.

Probably the most widely-discussed cost of the duty, however, is that stressed by Stone, who argues that imposition of a duty to warn will ultimately disadvantage the general public, potential patients, and actual patients. If therapists are saddled with a duty to warn potential victims, he asserts, therapists will be more reluctant—or completely unwilling—to treat patients who might give rise to the duty. Furthermore, the reduced confidentiality that can be promised potentially dangerous patients who are accepted for therapy will reduce the effectiveness of the therapy provided (6). To this might be added the danger that potentially dangerous patients might be discouraged from seeking therapy in the first place. The end result, in any case, will be that persons who pose significant dangers to others (and thus indirectly to themselves) will receive treatment less often, and the treatment they do receive will be less effective. Consequently, the danger which they pose will be increased because of the absence of available treatment opportunities.

Whether these costs will materialize is a factual question about which speculation is difficult. There is evidence that imposition of a duty to warn will affect therapists. Wise's study of California therapists after *Tarasoff* found that 54% of the therapists responding reported that after *Tarasoff* they experienced more anxiety when indications of dangerousness arose during therapy (3). To what extent, if any, this caused them to turn away potential patients because they perceived those potential patients as possibly dangerous was not investigated. Nor is there useful information available on the impact of the duty to warn on therapy. To some extent, the anti-therapeutic effects feared by Stone might be minimized if patients were not routinely told by the therapist at the beginning of therapy that the therapist might have to breach confidentiality by warning a possible victim. On the other hand, the existence of a duty to warn and its effect upon confidentiality might become generally known and affect potential and actual patients even if it is never the subject of discussion with the therapist. Wise concludes that *Tarasoff* did affect the substance of therapy provided by at least some California practitioners and that this change was "potentially detrimental" to the therapy. Some therapists responding to Wise's survey reported directing therapy more toward the possible assaultiveness of their patients; others reported concentrating on matters other than indications of possible dangerousness. While this information is useful, it is far from conclusive. We simply do not know whether fears such as those expressed by Stone are realistic.

CONCLUSION

The California Supreme Court's decision in *Tarasoff* has been widely misread. It does not create anything that can reasonably be regarded as a "duty to warn." Rather, it holds that in regard to identifying dangerous patients and reacting to the risk they pose to others, therapists will be held to the usual malpractice standard, which demands that they exercise the skill and care of their profession. Only if a failure to warn a potential victim, considered in light of all factors, constitutes a violation of this standard of care, will the therapist be liable for any harm caused to the victim by the patient.

The decision's holding that persons other than the patient could sue a therapist for a failure to exercise reasonable professional care does represent a significant expansion of liability, but other courts will probably be willing to take this same step if asked to do so. Once the right of third persons to sue therapists on the basis of professional negligence is acknowledged, application of the standard malpractice rule—as was done in *Tarasoff*— will be quite attractive to courts. At least one other appellate court has demonstrated this (17). Perhaps the most curious matter is that more courts have not yet addressed the third party issue.

How one evaluates the conflicting arguments regarding *Tarasoff*-type liability depends in part upon the available alternatives. There are several that require consideration. One would be continued adherence to the traditional position under which a therapist owes no duty to persons other than his or her patients. Under this state of affairs, no duty would be owed to potential victims, and so it would be unnecessary to consider how such a duty might be violated. Although this is the traditional position, it seems unlikely to be sufficiently attractive to find many judicial adherents in the future. Therapists' responsibilities to the public and even to specific third persons is too generally accepted to permit this solution. Even Stone acknowledges that therapists have—and should have—a moral duty to third persons, and that this is appropriately made a legal as well as a moral requirement (6).

Another possibility would be to recognize that therapists owe potential victims a duty of reasonable care, which requires that they exercise professional competence in identifying dangerous patients and taking steps to avoid injury to potential victims. This position would, however, be supplemented by a specific caveat that reasonable care never *requires* a warning or direct contact between the therapist and a potential victim. Discharge of the duty, in other words, could be adequately performed by seeking commitment or notifying law enforcement officers. This is one of the positions favored by Stone (6).

This alternative does not deal with the alleged unfairness of imposing upon therapists a duty to identify dangerous patients. It does, however, eliminate one of the major objections to such a duty and would perhaps remove much of the objectionable uncertainty created by such a duty. But in light of what seems to be more than negligible professional sentiment favoring the proposition that direct warnings are sometimes professionally acceptable and necessary, it seems an arbitrary fiat. Perhaps the matter is so fluid that, under a duty to warn, never or almost never will the failure to warn constitute action beyond the bounds of professional acceptability if some alternative action is taken. If so, the result would be the same. Given the uncertainty, it seems soundest to leave open the possibility that in some situations only a warning to the potential victim constitutes a professionally acceptable response to a dangerous patient.

A third possibility addresses the duty to identify dangerous patients rather than the duty to deal with the danger they pose. Stone has proposed that therapists should have a duty to third persons only when the therapist has actually made a determination that a patient is dangerous. Litigation would then be possible only when the therapist had acknowledged during consultation with a colleague or noted in the records that he/she had determined the patient to be dangerous. Suit could not be brought on the grounds that the therapist should have identified the patient as dangerous but did not (6).

This view also seems arbitrary. It might well discourage honest record-keeping or consultation, both of which seem to be quite desirable. Further, it assumes that the development of articulated criteria for identification of dangerous patients is either undesirable or impossible. Perhaps this is an illusory goal, but it seems too early to give up. On balance, there seems to be insufficient reason to single out the identification of dangerous patients as the unique area where therapists will not be held to an objective, reasonable, and professional standard.

What of the future? There is little reason to expect that the behavior of courts is any more predictable than that of patients in therapy, but it is an acceptable guess that other courts will find the *Tarasoff* result attractive and will follow it. The absence of many post-*Tarasoff* decisions, of course, attests to the relative rarity of such litigation, and it is unlikely that the near future will see a flood of it. It is, however, significant that a New Jersey trial judge was recently faced with the issue and, in the absence of controlling state law, chose to follow the *Tarasoff* result (17). As in *Tarasoff*, the matter was raised by a challenge to the plaintiff's pleadings, so the court's decision does not address the question of whether, on the facts of the particular case, the therapist's failure to warn the victim gave rise to liability. But it seems more likely than not that other courts will follow the same lead and permit plaintiffs—at least those able to support their position with expert testimony—to obtain a jury evaluation of whether a therapist is liable for damages because of a failure to warn the potential victim of the therapist's patient.

REFERENCES

1. Murderer Sues Psychiatrist for Not Preventing Crime. Austin (Texas) *American Statesman*, July 26, 1979, p. A11.
2. *Tarasoff v. Board of Regents*, 17 Cal. 3d 425, 131 Cal. Rptr. 14, 551 P.2d 334 (1976).
3. Wise, T. P.: Where the Public Peril Begins: A Survey of Psychotherapists to Determine the Effects of Tarasoff. *Stanford Law Review* 31:165-190, 1978.
4. Leonard, J. B.: A Therapist's Duty to Protect Victims, A Nonthreatening View of Tarasoff. *Law & Human Behavior*, 1:309-317, 1977.
5. Roth, L. H. and Meisel, A.: Dangerousness, Confidentiality, and the Duty to Warn. *Am. J. Psychiatry*, 134:508-511, 1977.
6. Stone, A. A.: The Tarasoff Decisions: Suing Psychotherapists to Safeguard Society. *Harvard Law Review*, 90:358-378, 1976.
7. Wexler, D. B.: Patients, Therapists, and Third Parties: The Victimological Virtues of Tarasoff. *International J. Law and Psychiatry*, 2:1-28, 1979.
8. Griffith, E. J. and Griffith, E. E. H.: Duty to Third Parties, Dangerousness, and the Right to Refuse Treatment: Problematic Concepts for Psychiatrist and Lawyer. *California Western Law Review*, 14:241-274, 1978.
9. Slovenko, R.: Psychotherapy and Confidentiality. *Cleveland State Law Review*, 24:375-396, 1975.
10. Principles of Medical Ethics With Annotations Especially Applicable to Psychiatry. *Am J. Psychiatry*, 130:1058-1064, 1973.
11. Fleming, J. G., and Maximov, B.: The Patient or His Victim: The Therapist's Dilemma. *California Law Review*, 62:1025-1068, 1974.
12. Meisel, A.: The "Exceptions" to the Informed Consent Doctrine: Striking

a Balance Between Competing Values in Medical Decisionmaking. Wisconsin Law Review 1979:413-488, 1979.

13. Waltz, J. R. and Scheuneman, T. W. Informed Consent to Therapy. *Northwestern U. Law Review*, 64:628-650, 1970.

14. Stone, A. A.: *Mental Health and Law: A System in Transition.* Washington: National Institute of Mental Health, 1975.

15. Kozol, H. L., Boucher, R. J., and Garofalo, R. F.: The Diagnosis and Treatment of Dangerousness. *Crime and Delinquency*, 18:371-392, 1972.

16. Monahan, J.: *The Prediction of Violent Criminal Behavior: A Methodological Critique and Prospectus, in Deterrence and Incapacitation: Estimating the Effects of Criminal Sanctions on Crime Rates.* Washington: National Academy of Sciences, 1978.

17. *McIntosh v. Milano,* 168 N.J. Super. 466, 403 A.2d 500 (1979).

18. Holbrook, J. T.: Psychotherapy and the Duty to Warn: A Tragic Trilogy: II. *Baylor Law Review,* 27:695-705, 1975.

19. Monahan, J.: Prediction Research and the Emergency Commitment of Dangerous Mentally Ill Persons: A Reconsideration. *Am J. Psychiatry,* 135:198-201, 1978.

Part III

THE PSYCHIATRIST AS AN EXPERT WITNESS

6

The Psychiatrist as Expert Witness

Richard T. Rada, M.D.

Recent social, political, and legal developments have broadened the interface between psychiatry and the law and have increased the likelihood that the individual psychiatrist will become involved in one way or another in the legal process. It is not necessary to document that psychiatrists serve as expert witnesses in the courtroom. The media delight in presenting a blow-by-blow description of the "battle of the experts," when psychiatrists are asked to testify in highly publicized criminal cases. What may be less well-known is that psychiatric consultation appears to be rapidly expanding in civil proceedings, including tort liability, workers' compensation, civil commitment, child custody, malpractice, and the like (1). The purpose of this essay is to discuss the role and preparation of the psychiatric expert witness as well as potential pitfalls of expert testimony, including countertransference issues.

THE LIMITED ROLE OF THE EXPERT WITNESS

A general principle of law is that courts have a right to every person's evidence and that the law gives the court the power to summon anyone to testify, except the President, and, as a rule, to compel that person to answer any question (2). When subpoenaed to court, the psychiatrist may be expected to serve in one of several capacities (3, 4).

The psychiatrist may be called as an ordinary citizen to report on witnessed facts. In these instances, special expertise is irrelevant to the testimony that is sought, and the witness is considered nonexpert.

The psychiatrist may also be called as a medical fact witness. In such cases, he/she may be asked to testify to certain medical facts regarding contact with a specific patient. For example, a psychiatrist who has seen a patient in consultation following an auto accident may be asked to state the presenting complaints, the findings on examination, the number of times the patient was seen, the fees for service, and the recommendations to the patient. The psychiatrist is expected to give factual answers but is not asked for opinions about these facts. He/she should, however, be aware that in certain jurisdictions the judge may require a medical fact witness to give an opinion, in which case the witness is first qualified as an expert and then asked for opinions. The likelihood of this possibility should always be discussed with a lawyer prior to appearance in court.

The psychiatrist may be called as an expert witness when both the facts and the conclusions to be drawn from them require professional and scientific knowledge or skill not within the ordinary range of knowledge and training of the average person. The privilege of testifying to both facts and opinions is peculiar to those deemed to be experts. Therefore, those called as potential expert witnesses must indicate by citing their special training, experience, knowledge, and skills that they have the qualifications of an expert. When psychiatrists are first called to testify in court, they sometimes balk at reciting all of their training and experience, professional affiliations, authorship of papers in professional journals, teaching and professional appointments, and the like, believing that this exercise is vain puffery and contrary to proper professional decorum. The witness' qualifications are, however, necessary not only to establish his/her status as an expert witness but also to help the jury evaluate the weight to be given to the testimony rendered. The judge determines who will be qualified as an expert. In fact, in most jurisdictions, the only essential qualification necessary to be declared an expert witness is proper licensure to practice medicine.

The psychiatrist may agree to serve as an expert for one side or the other in a dispute or, in some instances, may be appointed by the judge as an impartial expert witness for the court. When the expert agrees to testify on behalf of a client, it is understood that this testimony will aid that client. However, given the adversarial system of jurisprudence practiced in this country, there is not complete agreement on the manner in which the expert should present opinions in the courtroom. Some believe that the expert witness should strongly advocate opinions and conclusions, while others recommend a nonpartisan stance when testifying. Regardless of one's position on this question, all agree that the expert owes truth, fact, and accuracy to the cause of justice.

In recent years, the use of court-appointed impartial or neutral expert witnesses has received increased attention. The judge appoints a psychiatrist as an expert, who is charged with examining a particular client and submitting the findings to the court. This report is then given to the opposing attorneys. It is hoped that this approach will help assure impartiality, increase the likelihood that psychiatrists will agree to serve as expert witnesses, and allow for a more complete exposition of the expert's findings in the case. In some jurisdictions, the routine use of psychiatrists as impartial experts is reported to be effective (5). On the other hand, lawyers and psychiatrists have questioned the premise that experts called in this manner are truly impartial, and they assert that the use of a neutral witness only disguises the bias which the individual expert brings to his/her understanding of the case. What is most pertinent to this discussion is the common misperception that serving as an impartial witness eliminates the cross-examination. This is fiction. The facts and opinions of the impartial expert may be subjected in court to the same scrutiny as those presented by partisan experts (6).

The potential expert witness must understand not only the prerogatives but also the limits of the expert witness role. This seems self-evident, but it is surprising how often psychiatrists' dissatisfaction with serving as experts stems from a misperception of their proper role in the courtroom proceeding.

First, the expert witness is not the judge. In our country, a very elaborate and complicated body of rules of evidence has been established for the purpose of assuring a fair trial. It is for this reason that the question-and-answer format is used in a trial. The expert witness is not given free rein to state findings and opinions, as is more commonly the case in Europe. It is the judge's task to decide whether the questions asked of the expert will elicit facts and opinions relevant and material to the case. At times, an expert may feel stifled by a judge's ruling to limit certain aspects of his testimony. The judge, however, is the final arbiter and it is, at the very least, poor form to debate or question his/her decision. Nevertheless, many judges will allow expert witnesses at the end of their testimony to elaborate on opinions given in the direct or cross-examination.

Second, the expert witness is not the jury. It is the jury's task to decide what is "truth" in any particular case, even when that decision may conflict with the testimony rendered by an expert witness. Although each expert believes that his/her testimony is accurate, the jury must make the ultimate decision, which does not necessarily impeach or negate the validity of the expert's testimony. The most widely quoted example of this phenomenon is the Charlie Chaplin paternity case, in which Mr. Chaplin lost the paternity suit, even though expert medical testimony indicated that the blood types of the child and Mr. Chaplin were incompatible with paternity (7). In the case, the jury may have decided on the more global issue of the best interests of the child, rather than on the specific issue of paternity.

A further technical but important point: The expert is not expected to answer the ultimate legal question in the particular case. The judge or jury decide whether the facts and opinions lead to a particular conclusion, such as guilty or not guilty by reason of insanity. Although psychiatric expert witnesses may have formed opinons about the legal question, they are not expected to offer these opinions, and, if asked for these opinions, will frequently find that the opposing attorney will object to their answering.

Third, the expert witness is not the lawyer. Each attorney presents the evidence which is most likely to lead to a beneficial outcome for his/her client. To that end, the attorney will elicit from the expert those facts and opinions deemed most advantageous to the case. It is understood that experts will defend their conclusions under cross-examination, but they should refrain from subtly pleading the case by denying the possibility of other interpretations of the facts or by inappropriately arguing the merits of the case. Again, most judges will allow experts to qualify answers given to simplistically phrased yes or no type questions. When expert witnesses believe that they have not been able to present all of the facts and opinions in the case, the fault lies not with the opposing attorney but with a failure of proper communication between the experts and the attorney who has called them.

PREPARING TO SERVE AS AN EXPERT WITNESS

The importance of proper preparation for testifying as an expert witness cannot be overestimated. As in other areas of our professional training, the psychiatrist should consider the attitudinal, cognitive, and skill requirements for serving as an expert witness.

Attitudinal Preparation

The courtroom scene tends to arouse intense anxiety about a dreaded encounter rather than exhilaration about participation in a lofty and noble task. As I recently concluded a series of seminars on forensic psychiatry, one of the psychiatric residents turned to me and said: "We have found these discussions very interesting and stimulating and have decided to refer all of our court cases to you!" I will not, therefore, pretend to be overly sanguine or pollyannaish about ways to induce a positive attitude toward serving as an expert witness. Although the exact details may not be known, almost every psychiatrist is aware of those notorious instances in which a distinguished and eminent psychiatrist has ventured into the courtroom, only to leave feeling humiliated and degraded. One does not have to be arrogant, unwilling to have one's views questioned, as is often suggested by our legal colleagues, to feel threatened about courtroom testimony. The book, *Cross-Examination,* by trial practitioner John Appleman has the following revealing chapter subtitles: "Break Your Witness," "Step-by-Step Attack," "Witness on the Run," "Setting Traps for Opposing Counsel," "The Kill," "Shock Treatment," and "Discrediting Witnesses on Unimportant Matters" (8). The prospect of such treatment can be expected to influence even the most stout-hearted. Added to this are the frequent attacks from inside and outside the profession about the certitude of conclusions drawn from psychiatric observations and the social and moral discrediting of psychiatrists themselves. As Dietz has recently pointed out, "It is no wonder that psychiatrists perceive themselves as being under attack in an era in which their discreditors are cited as authority in briefs for the courts" (9).

The following are some suggestions for preparing yourself attitudinally for testifying in court:

1) Recognize that testifying in court is a serious matter and likely to produce anxiety in even the most experienced witness. The courtroom drama is, after all, expected to be serious, and the cause of truth and justice is not thought to be advanced by an informal and relaxed atmosphere. The witness stand is so termed because in the past (and occasionally in the present) the witness was made to stand while giving testimony. It was felt that allowing the witness to sit, and in some instances even to have water, was less likely to produce honest, straightforward testimony.

2) Rid yourself of the notion that you are above criticism because you are the expert. Overcome any feeling that you are infallible in your field.

3) Be prepared to act courteously even if subjected to improper treatment by opposing counsel. Although opposing counsel is entitled to a rigorous examination of the expert's qualifications,

findings, and conclusions, personal harassment and attack are improper. If the expert remains courteous during such attacks, the judge will frequently intervene and demand proper decorum from the attorney.

4) Recognize what we all know, but frequently forget in the courtroom, that we deal with issues which are not black or white. In preparing for courtroom testimony, objectively assess the strength of your conclusions. It is understood that not every conclusion is reached with the same level of confidence. Do not, therefore, allow yourself to be placed in the position of presenting each conclusion with equal certainty. Also be prepared to say, "I don't know," just as one would in any other professional situation.

5) No expert witness likes to be surprised by new facts presented by the opposing attorney at the trial. The best defense against this is a complete and thorough examination. The expert should, however, be open-minded about professional conclusions, and it is not personally discrediting for an expert to indicate that his/her conclusions might be altered by facts which were previously unavailable.

Cognitive Preparation

The recently established American Board of Forensic Psychiatry attests that the body of knowledge required by forensic psychiatrists is large enough to designate the field as a subspecialty. It has now become almost impossible to keep up with the field, and some forensic psychiatrists have already begun to specialize in areas such as criminal law, civil law, training, and research. Serving as an expert witness does not require an extensive knowledge of the total field, but there are several basic issues which the psychiatrist should consider.

A common and embarrassing situation for the expert witness is to have carefully prepared psychiatric testimony, only to find that he/she has addressed legal questions totally irrelevant to the particular case. An obvious example is the difference between the legal understanding of competency to stand trial and that of criminal responsibility at the time of the commission of the offense. Whenever asked to testify, the psychiatrist should immediately establish which legal questions will need to be addressed. Having carefully established this, any of the standard psychiatric textbooks on psychiatry and the law can be used as references to become informed about the specifics of the legal questions involved.

The statutes pertaining to civil and criminal proceedings vary from state to state. The prospective expert witness and the lawyer should meet and discuss the specific state statutes which apply to the legal questions which will be addressed in the particular case. Thus, in regard to criminal responsibility, over 20 states now use the American Law Institute's standard for determining criminal responsibility, while in other states the well known M'Naghten rule is still used. In a few states a combination of M'Naghten and the "irresistible impulse" is the legal standard. In such jurisdictions, failure to attend to both of these questions is not only embarrassing for expert witnesses but also tends to nullify their testimony, however effective it may be when applied to only one of the legal requirements.

It is often erroneously assumed that standards for legal questions and statutory law are written in a very precise and exact method (10). Quite the opposite is generally true. There can be considerable differences of opinion regarding the meaning of legal terms such as "malice," "negligence," and "substantial capacity." Unless competent as a forensic specialist, the psychiatrist must rely on the attorney to clarify the legal understanding of the various terms. For example, I recently testified in a case in which a significant portion of the testimony hinged on the definition of the word "deliberation," and, in this case, the prosecution and the defense each understandably chose a definition of the word which would be most advantageous to his/her own side. Having thoroughly researched with the attorney the different interpretations of the word, I was not placed in the position of unwittingly contradicting myself but was able to apply the facts and psychiatric conclusions to the two different definitions offered by the opposing attorneys.

Proper cognitive preparation does not require that the expert witness become an amateur lawyer. What is required is a basic understanding of those legal questions to which the psychiatric findings apply.

Skill Preparation

Proper and effective courtroom testimony requires skill that is acquired through practice. It is a curious fact that generally prudent, careful, and thoughtful psychiatrists will yield to the temptation to testify in highly publicized, complex legal cases, often with predictable results. It is good advice for the beginner, no matter how prestigious his/her reputation in the field, to start slowly and with less controversial legal cases.

Select cases carefully. Before taking a case, thoroughly discuss and clarify the relevant psychiatric issues. If, for example, the case relates to important questions about organic brain syndromes, and this is not the potential witness' area of expertise, referral to a colleague with more experience in that area might be advisable. The simple rule is to take cases in which your expertise is most pertinent.

Pretrial practice in presenting testimony, especially in answering the likely cross-examination questions, can be invaluable. Most attorneys are quite willing to meet with the psychiatrist and conduct a practice examination on the issues in the case.

If psychiatrists start slowly, accept cases which come within their knowledge and expertise, and adequately prepare for the case with the attorney, they will be rewarded with the personal satisfaction of knowing that their skill in testifying will increase with each case.

THE PITFALLS OF TESTIFYING

Much has been written about the importance of specific details in psychiatric expert testimony, including proper courtroom etiquette and strategies for dealing with the cross-examination (3). I would now like to emphasize two areas which are not sufficiently addressed by other sources.

The Uninformed Participant

1) *The psychiatrist.* In the preceding section on preparation of the expert witness, I focused on the broad areas of attitudinal, cognitive, and skill preparation. All of these are important, but nothing is, in my opinion, more important than familiarity with all the details of the specific case requiring testimony. For example, extensive handwritten notes or tape recordings of contacts with the clients can prove invaluable. The expert who trusts important and significant facts in the psychiatric history to memory invites a very detailed cross-examination.

Insist on a pretrial meeting with the attorney to discuss in detail the psychiatric findings, the legal questions to be asked, and the answers you intend to give. (It is a maxim of trial lawyers that one never asks a witness a question without knowing what the answers will be). Critically discuss weaknesses in the case, and consider those areas which are likely to be covered on cross-examination. Thorough pretrial preparation means that there will be fewer or no unexpected questions.

2) *The lawyer.* Do not assume that all lawyers are knowledgeable trial lawyers, and above all do not assume that each lawyer fully comprehends the legal issues involved in cases requiring psychiatric testimony. This can be a serious problem when both the lawyer and the psychiatrist are relatively inexperienced. Proper pretrial preparation can alert both parties to these deficiencies, and it is then essential that they establish a working relationship to correct for their knowledge deficiencies. Public defenders often have little time to prepare their cases because of their heavy workload. Likewise, many private attorneys do not spend a significant portion of their time in courtroom trials. As with any professional group, the lawyer may not have the most up-to-date knowledge about the particular area encompassed by the litigation. The psychiatrist has an obligation to teach and

inform the lawyer about the most effective means for obtaining the information. When presented in a nonarrogant manner, lawyers appreciate the advice of their expert witnesses regarding appropriate questions, timing of the questions, and strategies for dealing with likely cross-examination issues. Psychiatric testimony is most often rendered ineffective, not by a grilling cross-examination, but by an inept and unprepared direct examination by the lawyer who has called the psychiatric expert.

Countertransference Issues

Subtler than lack of preparation or anxiety about the cross-examination are the pitfalls which arise because of common countertransference reactions among expert witnesses. What follows is a discussion of the more common countertransference reactions and the sources from which they arise.

Sources of countertransference reactions include the legal system, the legal profession, the specific participants in the legal process, the clients, and colleagues, namely, the expert witness(es) for the opposing side.

The adversarial nature of the legal process runs counter to the beliefs and attitudes of most psychiatrists. The discipline of psychiatry is built on understanding and empathy for the views and opinions of others, and psychotherapy is frequently an attempt to promote appropriate intrapsychic and interpersonal communication and compromise. Thus, the adversarial system is not only foreign but, in some sense, antithetical to the psychiatrist's purpose. In addition, psychiatrists themselves may have been involved in legal proceedings such as divorce, child custody, or malpractice, whose outcome may have left a less than optimal feeling about the likelihood of justice being dispensed within the legal system.

Another source of countertransference stems from friction and hostility between the two professions. In recent years, members of the legal profession have been among the most strident critics of the field of psychiatry. Furthermore, psychiatrists undoubtedly share with the average person certain negative feelings toward the legal profession, attitudes which are attested to by practically all surveys measuring respect and regard for the various professions, surveys in which the legal profession often comes out at the bottom. Given the current interprofessional milieu, it is not unlikely that the psychiatrist will have certain unconscious, if not conscious, negative feelings about participating in the courtroom drama.

The legal professionals in a trial can evoke strong reactions within the psychiatrist. For example, the professional reputation of local judges is often well-known. The "hanging judge" is a specific case in point. When serving as a psychiatric expert witness for a defendant being tried by such a judge, there may be a tendency, conscious or unconscious, to skew the data in favor of the defendant. In addition to judges, lawyers have a powerful potential for evoking both positive and negative countertransference feelings. Even over the telephone, some lawyers (in my experience, unsure and inexperienced ones) may act in a hostile, arrogant, and demanding fashion. No one likes to be treated that way, but it is essential that expert witnesses do not allow these feelings to carry over into their dealings with the client or the conclusions based on their findings.

The litigants themselves, the patients or clients, can be another important source of countertransference feelings. Psychiatrists must be acutely aware of the potential for conflict when dealing with certain types of cases and certain types of defendants. Thus, child custody cases, sex offender cases (especially child molesters), and workers' compensation cases can be so heavily tinged with bias about the clients themselves that the psychiatrist's objectivity is seriously strained. Criminal defendants, in particular, present certain obvious problems. Despite intrapsychic resistances familiar to psychiatrists, most patients who seek psychiatric consultation attempt to be honest and open. The ability of sociopaths to con the average person, including psychiatrists, is well-known. It is, at the very least, disconcerting to be hoodwinked or misled by clients, especially when one is working in their behalf.

Reactions to the opposition's expert witness(es) must not be underestimated. Sibling rivalry issues among psychiatric expert witnesses are not unknown, sometimes rationalized or thinly disguised by labeling the other expert "a hired gun." Experienced expert witnesses know that the conclusion of a case involving a "battle of the experts" cannot be attributed solely to the truth, value, or strength of the expert testimony. Nevertheless, it is far easier to walk out of a courtroom unconcerned about the final outcome when one is the only expert appearing. This often becomes more difficult when one is appearing in opposition to a colleague. Sibling rivalry is sometimes aided and abetted by the lawyers themselves. I recently served as a consultant for a rape case in which the district attorney based much of his presentation on material taken from work I had published. Following the case, he called to thank me for my advice but added in closing that, while cross-examining the defendant's expert witness, a colleague of mine, he had asked the witness if he considered Dr. Rada an authority in the field of rape. I realized that it was wise, when serving as an expert, not to give carte blanche recognition to anyone's authority, because that authority's work can then be quoted in opposition to one's own opinions. I was not surprised, therefore, to learn that this experienced witness had indicated that he did not consider me to be an authority. I must admit, however, that the thought crossed my mind of asking him at the next cocktail party whether his denial of my expertise in the field was useful courtroom strategy, or based on real ignorance.

Having considered the major sources of countertransference reactions, we may now turn to the more common reactions experienced by expert witnesses.

Overadvocacy is, in my opinion, the most common countertransference reaction. As mentioned previously, some authorities believe that the expert should never take an advocacy position. I do not share this view. Having arrived at conclusions as objectively as possible, the expert should, in a firm, confident manner, advocate his/her views in the courtroom. However, overadvocacy characterized either by stubborn refusal to admit fallibility or histrionic pleading of the case is out of place in the courtroom.

It is true that a tendency to overadvocacy is sometimes a response to the courtroom situation itself. At an inquest, even scientific evidence may be presented cautiously. By the time the evidence is to be presented at trial, however, opinions tend to solidify as a result of the courtroom proceedings and also because the type of questioning from both sides often appreciates, if it does not demand, a certainty which is greater than may be the intent, desire, or knowledge of the expert witness.

Although the demand characteristics of the courtroom situation often lead to overadvocacy, identification with the client is the likeliest source. The circumstances which bring people into the courtroom are often tragic, and even in cases involving assault and murder, the psychiatrist comes not only to understand the dynamics of the offense but often to feel empathy or sympathy for the defendant. Sometimes there is a sense of identification with the underdog, especially in criminal cases where the individual lacks the social support system to counter what often seems the immense power of the criminal justice system.

Excessive hostility is the reaction most often noted and discussed by lawyers when evaluating physician expert witnesses (11). Feelings of hostility are understandable when, as is unfortunately sometimes the case, the expert witness is treated discourteously or frankly harassed. But the source of most hostile responses in expert witnesses stems, in my opinion, from a sense of insecurity about the facts in the case and about their role as expert witnesses. It is always a pleasure to testify about competency or criminal responsibility when the evidence for the client's mental illness follows textbook descriptions. Unfortunately, few offenders conform to the textbooks, and expert witnesses must frequently formulate their opinions without the advantage of getting to know the patient intimately through repeated contact.

Occasionally the expert witness succumbs to identification with the aggressor, in this instance, the lawyer. It is probably true that many psychiatrists who engage in expert testimony find the law and the courtroom drama fascinating and appealing. In fact, some forensic psychiatrists are lawyers, teach in law schools, or have taken pertinent law school courses. Identification with the aggressor can lead to an argumentative, legalistic presentation of the findings by the expert. There is a fine line between presenting and advocating one's findings and conclusions and engaging in a debate with opposing counsel. Playing one-upmanship with opposing counsel rarely serves the best interest of the client. Another reaction, excessive humility, is quite rare, but, when it occurs, it has serious consequences for the client. Although experts should recognize and admit that they are not infallible, excessive humility about their own skills or the skills of the profession will be used by opposing attorneys to make the experts appear waffling, incompetent, and unsure of the basis of their conclusions. Excessive humility can afflict both very inexperienced and very distinguished and highly regarded psychiatrists. In the latter instance, the distinguished psychiatrist may feel that his/her reputation should carry the day and therefore may not present findings with the straightforward assurance and certitude that is necessary to have a proper impact on the jury.

CONCLUSION

Serving as an expert witness does not appeal to all psychiatrists. Unfortunately, the reluctance of experienced psychiatrists to testify in court deprives clients and the court of some of the best and most up-to-date knowledge that our profession has to offer. With careful and thorough preparation and attention to the common pitfalls, the psychiatrist can render a true service to the community as an expert witness and can, to quote Henry Davidson, leave the courtroom with his "face and veracity intact" (12).

REFERENCES

1. Sadoff, R. L.: The expanding role of psychiatric consultation in civil-legal proceedings. In: C. H. Wecht, (Series Ed.) *Legal Medicine Annual: Nineteen Seventy.* New York: Appleton-Century-Crofts, 1970.
2. Slovenko, R.: *Psychiatry and Law.* Boston: Little, Brown & Company, 1973.
3. Davidson, H. A.: *Forensic Psychiatry,* Second Edition. New York: Ronald Press Company, 1965.
4. Waltz, J. R. and Inbau, F. E.: *Medical Jurisprudence.* New York: Macmillan Publishing Co., 1971.

5. Aring, C. D. Expert medical testimony. *Journal of the American Medical Association*, 236:569, 1976.
6. Moenssens, A. A.: "Impartial" medical experts: New look at an old issue. In: C. H. Wecht, (Series Ed.) *Legal Medicine Annual: Nineteen Seventy-Four*. New York: Appleton-Century-Crofts, 1974.
7. *Berry v. Chaplin*, 74 Ca. App. 2d 562, 169 p.2d 442 (1946).
8. Appleman, J. A.: *Cross-examination*. Fairfax, Va.: Coiner Publications, 1963.
9. Dietz, P. E.: Social discrediting of psychiatry: The protasis of legal disfranchisement. *Am. J. Psychiat.*, 134:1356-1360, 1977.
10. Slovenko, R.: Reflections on the criticisms of psychiatric expert testimony. *Wayne Law Rev.*, 25:37-66, 1978.
11. Caruso, P.: The most hostile, hostile witness—the doctor. *Medical Trial Technique Quarterly*, 19:241-245, 1973.
12. Davidson, H. A. On being cross-examined. *Am. J. Psychiat.*, 106:424-428, 1949.

7

Psychological Testimony and Presumptions in Child Custody Cases

Ralph Slovenko, LL.B., Ph.D.

Family breakups have presented the law with a new kind of dispute. When the family was the basic economic unit, divorce was rare, and problems of child custody almost nonexistent. Now that the corporation or (in some places) the commune has replaced the extended family as the economic unit, there are fewer ties holding the family together. The family may stay together or separate now for emotional reasons. Succinctly put: "First we were an extended family, then we were a nuclear family, and now we're divorced" (1).

The new no-fault divorce law is a factor contributing to more child-custody litigation. Under the old fault-ground law, a husband wanting a divorce would be inclined to accept a settlement on support and child custody in exchange for the decree. This bargaining usually occurred where proof of misconduct was lacking, but one or both parties had enough of the marriage. Under the no-fault law, the husband, assured of divorce, is less inclined to agree in advance to the wife's demands regarding child custody and property matters. The husband today often asks for child custody as a means to extort a settlement or reduce an unfair demand made by the wife. This tactic may be the only weapon in his legal arsenal.

Under the old divorce law, the parents often arrived at an accommodation as to property settlement, alimony, support, and custody, which was presented to the court for approval. One of them then withdrew from the lawsuit, permitting the judge to grant the divorce without an actual contested trial. Under no-fault, however, the parties, anticipating that they will receive their divorce, are often unwilling to make concessions, particularly on property settlements, and more cases reach the trial stage. (When actually granted custody, one husband of an acquaintance exclaimed to his lawyer, "I got custody? You fool!") Ironically, no-fault divorce, although aimed at alleviating disputes, has resulted in more contests in family matters. It typifies legislation that produces results contrary to those actually desired.

This is not to say that a custody dispute arises in every case of divorce where there are children. In the majority of cases, divorce is uncontested and raises no custody problem. As a rule, the father recognizes that the mother can provide better care and the children wish to be with the mother. Consequently, the father does not request child custody or possession of the family home in the divorce action, or he does so only to have some bargaining leverage. (More often, the actual dispute is over possession and maintenance of the automobile.) While there are fathers who are single-minded about obtaining custody (2), most realize that a custody trial is likely to be an expensive and futile endeavor. Maternal custody is awarded in over 90% of the contested cases.

In the days when divorce was exceptional, the fundamental principle in family law was that the father possessed the paramount right to the custody and control of his minor children. When divorce scarcely existed, the father was in control, but as the mother was the center of the home, she was *de facto* though not *de jure* the custodian. The mother's legal right to custody of her children was recognized only on the death of the father.

The issue of custodianship, when it arose, usually involved a relative or other third person who sought custody of the child to prevent parental neglect or abuse. Courts invariably held for the natural parent, on the theory that the child was the property of the parent.

With the emancipation of women, and the growing incidence of divorce, a parental-right doctrine could hardly resolve custody disputes between parents. Beginning with Justice Cardozo's decision in 1925 in *Finlay v. Finlay* (3), the courts have come to say that the prime consideration in child-custody disputes is the best interests of the child. In application, the best-interest test is usually a parental-right decision. In a *parent v. parent* contest, the mother obtains custody in the vast majority of cases. In a *parent v. non-parent* contest, the child's best interest is usually said to be custody by the parent. This fusion of the best-interest and parental-right doctrines stems from the view that custody by a natural parent, particularly the mother, is in the best interest of the child. The Commissioners' comment to the Uniform Marriage and Divorce Act states that: "The preference for the mother as custodian of young children when all things are equal . . . is simply a shorthand method of expressing the best interest of children" (4). This language was cited recently by the Kentucky Supreme Court in overruling a lower court award of custody of a young child to the father (5).

The phrase "best interests of the child" is magnanimous, but what criteria or evidence do the courts use in reaching such a decision? The principle is not used to bar a divorce, though in a great many—perhaps most—cases a divorce is contrary to the best interests of the children. It is not in the best interest of the child to be without both parents at home (except in extreme cases), or to be shuttled from one parent to the other. When the family breaks apart, without other support, the child tends to lose his sense of security and to feel that he has been abandoned by the noncustodial parent (6). The best-interest principle, however, is invoked only *after* the granting of divorce, nowadays available for the asking.

In ordinary litigation, the individuals most immediately affected by the dispute participate in the adjudicatory process, but in a child custody dispute, the child, legally speaking, is not a party in the process. Though the doctrine in child custody disputes may be the "best interests of the child," the child does not have representation in the ordinary sense, and does not define these interests himself. A number of lawyers and mental health professionals have recently argued that the child's interest in custody litigation would be best served by a child advocate (7). A number of states have adopted the recommendation of the Uniform Marriage and Divorce Act that "the court may appoint an attorney to represent the interests of a minor or dependent child with respect to his custody, support, and visitation" (8). But what will the child's attorney advocate? The traditional role of the lawyer is to advise and advocate the client's express desires. He looks to the client for guidance and instruction, but in a custody dispute a child's representative, except in the case of older children, must himself define the child's interests (9). Moreover, since the child is not, by law, a party to the dispute, he has no right of appeal. Many states now require a judge to consider the preference of the child in applying the best-interests standard; the preference of young persons older than 12 or 14 is by statute in some states made determinative or highly dispositive of the issue.

A frequently advanced contention is that formulation of custody standards and custody decision-making would be enhanced by psychological learning. In 1963, a commentator in the *Yale Law Journal* argued: "Optimum custody goals [of the best interests of the child standard] may be further defined by concentration on the psychological well-being of the child, where 'psychological well-being' is used to denote the mental and emotional health of the child—specifically, a process of personality development within the framework of patterns of normal growth as posited by the behavioral sciences" (10). In this seminal article, the author argued that courts should adopt a "psychological best interests test" (11). "Inquiry should be made into the fundamental relationship between 'psychological' parent and child" (12). Under a psychological best-interests test, "[the] primary aim would be to identify and describe the existing affection-relationship(s), chiefly from the perspective of the particular child who is the subject of the custody dispute. Such relationships might be inferred from evidence shedding light on three questions: the continuity of the relationship between child and adult in terms of proximity and duration; the love of the adult toward the child; and the affection and trust of the child toward the adult" (13).

In 1968, Joseph Goldstein, a law professor and psychoanalyst (later to co-author *Beyond the Best Interests of the Child*), wrote in the *Yale Law Journal*: "If the law student (who is also hopefully the future judge) were to study the primary sources of psychoanalysis, he would see that at most and at best a psychoanalytically-informed definition of the child's best interests would assist court or adoption agency in deciding which disposition among available alternatives is likely to provide the child, whatever his endowments, with the best available opportunity to fulfill his potential in society as a civilized human being" (14). In the book, *Beyond the Best Interests of the Child,* published in 1973, Goldstein together with Anna Freud and A. J. Solnit suggested that legal standards were giving too little consideration to the psychological well-being of the child. They proposed "generally applicable guidelines" to govern all child placement disputes. These guidelines would require a court to choose for a particular child the "least detrimental available alternative," which the authors defined as: "[T]hat child placement and procedure for child placement which maximizes, in accord with the child's sense of time . . . the child's opportunity for being wanted . . . and for maintaining on a continuous, unconditional, and permanent basis a relationship with at least one adult who is or will become the child's psychological parent" (15). Goldstein, Freud and Solnit defined a "psychological parent" as "one who, on a continuing day-to-day basis, through interaction, companionship, interplay, and mutuality, fulfills the child's psychological needs for a parent, as well as the child's physical needs" (16).

In the 1960s, there were a number of other statements on the psychological best interests of the child. Andrew Watson described, in a number of articles, various factors that would be relevant to the application of a psychological best interest of the child test (17). In 1967, the American Orthopsychiatric Association issued a position statement on child custody, following on the heels of the much publicized litigation in *Painter v. Bannister* (18). This case involved a contest between a father and maternal grandparents over the custody of a seven-year-old boy. The boy's mother was killed in an automobile accident, and the father asked the grandparents to take care of the boy. The father, when subsequently remarrying, wanted the boy back. The grandparents refused, and litigation ensued. The AOA's statement (formulated by Richard Jenkins, child psychiatrist) read as follows:

> The American Orthopsychiatric Association supports the view that the determining consideration in child custody cases should be the welfare of the child. Children are not property and should not be regarded as possessions. The rights of a parent to the custody of his child are dependent upon his assuming parental responsibility and functioning as a parent. While there is a strong initial presumption that the custody of a child should rest with his natural parent, the law has long recognized that this presumption may be set aside if the parent is unfit for or fails to assume parental responsibilities.
>
> The Association believes that the presumption in favor of the parent should rest upon the actual existence of a deep bond of mutual attachment between child and parent, such as normally grows out of a parent-child and child-parent relationship. Where such a bond exists, it outweighs all consideration of what advantages a foster home may have to offer because of wealth, education or social position. Within the range of lawful behavior it is more important than any value judgment about the family atmosphere. On the other hand, when the natural parent has not functioned as a parent, or has been so ineffectual in that functioning that no such mutual bond exists, and when a mutual bond has developed between the child and a foster parent, such a developed relation is, in the judgment of this Association, also worthy of a great respect in the determination of child custody.

In terms of the future mental health of our population, the welfare of the child, not the welfare nor interests of the parent nor of the foster parent, should be the determining consideration. This Association will study such issues as the kinds of criteria and evidence which should be useful in deciding what may be in the best interests of the child (19).

To have custody disputes determined by psychological and psychiatric theories requires analysis of the limits of these theories, their empirical bases, and the capacity of the legal system to absorb them. Consider, for example, a case where the father is very predictable, while the wife is artsy and emotional (20). Is the law to place the greater value on predictability or emotionality? How do these qualities affect the psychological best interests of the child? Professor Robert Mnookin asks:

> Can psychologists and psychiatrists consistently differen-tiate between a situation where an adult and a child have a substantial relationship of the sort we characterize as parent-child and that where there is no such relationship at all? Do existing psychological theories provide the basis to choose generally between two adults where the child has some relationship and psychological attachment to each? In cases where, from the child's perspective, each claimant has a psychological relationship with the child, do you think there would often be widespread consensus among experts about which parent would prove pyschologically better (or less detrimental) to the child? Often each parent will have a different sort of relationship with the child, with the child attached to each. One may be warm, easygoing, but in-capable of discipline. The other may be fair, able to set limits, but unable to express affection. By what criteria is an expert to decide which is less detrimental? Moreover, even the proponents of psychological standards have acknowl-edged how problematic it is to evaluate relationships from a psychological perspective unless a highly trained person spends a considerable amount of time observing the parent and child interact or talking to the child. Superficial exam-inations by those without substantial training may be worse than nothing. And yet, that is surely a high risk.
> Even with the best trained experts, would the choice

often be based on predictions that are beyond the demonstrated capacity for any existing theory? (21)

A negative view of psychological testing for deciding custody
cases has marked the literature. For example, Professor Sheila
Okpaku states:

> [P]sychology at this point is unable to supply the predic-
> tive assistance that courts need, [so] courts must recognize
> and accept the existing limitations on the ability to foresee
> the likely consequences of custody alternatives.
> [In easy custody cases,] the limitations on the ability to
> foresee the results of custody arrangements were of minimal
> significance because of the strength of cultural assumptions
> concerning desirable and undesirable child-rearing practices.
> Thus, a loving mother is virtually assured custody upon
> divorce just as a parent who has left the child with third
> parties for most of its formative years is virtually certain
> to be denied custody. In reaching such results, courts invoke
> the decisional guidelines which embody assumptions concern-
> ing blood ties, maternal love, and parental neglect. . . .
> [T]hese assumptions work less well in difficult cases because
> the latter present alternatives which are less clear-cut. It
> has also been noted that the predominant characteristic in
> difficult cases was their 'closeness'; no party had a clear claim
> to a preference under the prevailing decisional guidelines.
> Indeed . . . *either* result in a difficult case could be defended.
> . . . Until behavioral scientists demonstrate the special
> knowledge they sometimes claim, it is hoped that the pleas
> for the assistance of experts which punctuate opinions will
> be replaced by an informed skepticism concerning the present
> decisional utility of psychological testimony, and a more
> honest reliance on the experientially based discretion of trial
> judges (22).

Professor Areen in her "Family Law" casebook, used in a number of law schools, includes transcript material to illustrate
how little is gained from extensive use of expert witnesses on
fine points of distinction between two fit parents (23). D. W.
Winnicott, the respected English psychoanalyst, suggested an
"ordinary good parent" concept—that is, a "good enough parent"
should have full legal right to custody. This orientation would

eliminate the necessity of determining the psychologically "best" parent by a complicated formula drawn out by behavioral scientists (24).

The movement to formulate custody standards on the basis of psychology, however, is prevailing, and psychological evidence is playing an increasingly important role in custody disputes. The "psychological best interests test" opens the door to the mental health professional as expert (25). More and more, the psychiatrist, psychologist or social worker is called upon to testify. At the same time, investigators from the office of the "Friend of the Court" are routinely qualified by the court as experts. The educational requirements of these investigators vary considerably —some counties simply require a high school diploma, others emphasize experience, still others require advanced degrees in behavioral or social sciences. Some might suggest a preference for a child psychiatrist, and so at trial, the examiner might ask the expert if he is a child psychiatrist, implying that such an expert can best assess the best interests of the child. The teacher, though having extensive contact with the child, is rarely, if ever, called as a witness. The mental health professional is also given preference over friends or neighbors, not only because the latter tend to twist their story in favor of the parent of their liking but also because they cannot testify probatively on psychological best interest.

To what extent should the legal standards for the resolution of custody disputes be discretionary? Would hard or semihard rules be better? What substantive standards, if any, are to prevail in a custody case? Is each case instead to be decided on its own facts? One realizes that the fundamental precept of justice is that like cases should be decided alike. We proclaim that ours is a government of law, not of men (or loopholes). The precept that like decisions be given in like cases significantly limits the discretion of judges and others in authority (26). Does this precept make sense in custody cases, where it is said that no two cases are alike, and that no process is more fair than one requiring resolution in a highly individualized manner?

Professors Henry Foster and Doris Freed have observed that

nowhere has the task of achieving "a workable compromise between the values of flexibility and certainty . . . proved more challenging than in the area of child custody" (27). Some commentators have criticized the broad discretion granted judges, and they have suggested that rules are needed. For example, Phoebe C. Ellesworth and Robert J. Levy in their report prepared for the National Conference of Commissioners on Uniform State Laws recommended that the law should articulate a series of "presumptions" which under ordinary circumstances would relieve the judge of extensive fact-finding and decision-making responsibility, and, they say, would cut down on litigation (28). By "presumption," a substantive rule of law is intended which would mandate a particular custody disposition in the absence of strong rebutting testimony. For example, Ellesworth and Levy suggest that the law should contain a presumption favoring maternal custody—at least for young children, and probably for children of any age. It might be appropriate, for example, to permit the father to attempt to prove that the child has some special need which can only be satisfied if the father is named custodian. Ellesworth and Levy maintain, however, that it is essential that the standards be stated clearly and that the judge's role be simplified and substantially eased.

Thus, it has been considered that a mere instruction to the judge to be guided by the "best interests of the child" would be abstract and valueless (though it does shift the focus from parental rights to the child's interests). The recommendation of the Uniform Marriage and Divorce Act provides more elaborate instructions:

> The court shall determine custody in accordance with the best interest of the child. The court shall consider all relevant factors including:
>
> 1) the wishes of the child's parent or parents as to his custody;
> 2) the wishes of the child as to his custodian;
> 3) the interaction and interrelationship of the child with his parent or parents, his siblings, and any other person who may significantly affect the child's best interest;

4) the child's adjustment to his home, school, and community; and
5) the mental and physical health of all individuals involved.

The court shall not consider conduct of a proposed custodian that does not affect his relationship to the child (29).

Legislation has been enacted setting out criteria some of which have articulated presumptions. Michigan in its Child Custody Act of 1970, the first statute to set out the criteria of best interests of the child, defines "best interests of the child" as the sum total of designated factors to be considered, evaluated, and determined by the court:

(a) The love, affection, and other emotional ties existing between the competing parties and the child.
(b) The capacity and disposition of competing parties to give the child love, affection, and guidance, and continuation of the education and raising of the child in its religion or creed, if any.
(c) The capacity and disposition of competing parties to provide the child with food, clothing, medical care, or other remedial care recognized and permitted under the laws of this state in lieu of medical care, and other material needs.
(d) The length of time the child has lived in a stable, satisfactory environment and desirability of maintaining continuity.
(e) The permanence, as a family unit, of the existing or proposed custodial home.
(f) The moral fitness of the competing parties.
(g) The home, school, and community record of the child.
(h) The mental and physical health of the competing parties.
(i) The reasonable preference of the child, if the court deems the child to be of sufficient age to express preference.
(j) Any other factor considered by the court to be relevant to a particular child-custody dispute (30).

The Michigan legislation, which has served as a paradigm in other states, is thus replete with terms as elastic as a rubber band. Though the legislation purports to provide standards, the trial judge working under it has broad discretion in rendering a decision. The Michigan Act actually contains only one presumption, apart from the one giving weight to the "reasonable preference of the child if the court deems the child to be of sufficient age to express preference" (31). In another section of the Act, it is provided that there is a rebuttable presumption that the best interests of the child require that he should remain in the custody of a natural parent as against the claim of a third party. It states: "When the dispute is between the parents, between agencies, or between third persons, the best interests of the child shall control. When the dispute is between the parent or parents and an agency or a third person, it is presumed that the best interests of the child are served by awarding custody to the parent or parents unless the contrary is established by clear and convincing evidence" (32). The Act had another presumption favoring maternal custody in a *parent v. parent* dispute, but that was removed in a revision of the law in 1970; after all, today's mother is likely to be out working (33).

There seems to be a trend today arguing for legislation that would provide a presumption of joint custody as the preferred option, though the court already has the power to award joint custody under its statutory authority over the child (34). The advocates of joint custody seek an express legislative declaration of public policy stating that joint custody is to be encouraged, or that such an alternative must be given first consideration (35). There is, however, much debate over just what joint custody is. Presumably joint custody would give both parties, together or separately as in marriage, a voice in how the child is to be parented—for example, the child's education, residence, and medical care (36). But how will joint custody work as a practical matter? Will it work only when the parties get along? (In such cases, they do not need the order of a court.) Will it affect the mother's chances of remarriage? Will it create more instability, more shuttling, in the lives of children?

In a way, the joint custody presumption attempts to take the court out of family disputes, but in actuality, it will keep lawyers busy forever. Another move to take the court out of family disputes, though by an opposite route, is the recommendation that the judge should decide only who is to be parent, and not how the child is to be parented. Expressed differently, the judge is to restrict his activity to *who* shall have custody and not consider *how* or *under what conditions* the custodian and child are to relate to one another and to others. The one parent selected is to be relied upon entirely to respond to the child's ever-changing day-to-day needs. This autonomous parent would have absolute control over visitation as over other matters (37). (The presumption of parental autonomy resembles in a way the type of postdivorce situation prevailing, for example, in Poland, where husband usually remarries shortly after divorce, embarks on a new life and has no association with the children of his prior marriage; the mother is invariably given custody. One may find that, given the divorce, such an arrangement is in the best interests of the children.)

Under the Michigan Child Custody Act or similar legislation in other states, the criteria set out for determining the best interests of the child do not necessarily have to be weighed equally, but each must be addressed by one or more witnesses as the court is obliged to consider and make findings with respect to all of the factors described in the legislation (38). The sum total of these factors (not arithmetical, of course) is deemed to constitute the "best interests of the child," and, according to the law, must "control" the decision. Invariably, however, a "battle of the experts" takes place in custody disputes as to what is in the "best interests of the child." One may be reminded of a closing argument by a leading New York trial lawyer: "Experts! Experts! They are like asparagus. You buy them by the bunch!"

In child custody disputes, contradictory views are expressed, for example, on the merits of joint or alternating or divided custody, or on splitting the children. Contradictory opinions are also expressed on other questions: Are certain types of behavior so detrimental to a child's welfare that they should disqualify a parent as a custodian? Should a homosexual be denied custody or visitation rights (39)? Should the parents' or the child's wishes regarding custody be taken into consideration? Should the noncustodial parent have legal duties in terms of the child's welfare other than the payment of support? Should children be separated when one over the age of 12 or 14 expresses a desire to be with the father, leaving the younger with the mother? What are the advantages or disadvantages of choosing the mother, or of choosing the father (40)? Do they vary with the age or sex of the child? What are the effects of removing the child, temporarily during litigation or permanently, from both parents?

When push comes to shove, what actually are the major determinants in deciding custody? Robert Woody, a clinical psychologist, gleaned a list of 20 factors that had been mentioned in lawbooks through the years as guiding decisions about child custody, and he asked professionals to rank-order them. In his book, "*Getting Custody/Winning the Last Battle of the Marital War,*" Woody sets out these 20 factors concerning parents in order of importance as follows: 1) quality of relationship with the child; 2) mental health; 3) child-rearing attitudes; 4) child-care history; 5) personal history; 6) physical health; 7) general life history; 8) personality; 9) morality; 10) criminal record; 11) intelligence; 12) income; 13) knowledge of child development; 14) stability of residence; 15) education; 16) aspirations; 17) age; 18) sexual behavior; 19) religion; and 20) vocation (41). When one reviews court cases, however, it is obvious that the sex of the parent is the primary determinant. The factors mentioned above come into play only in the exceptional case, where the mother (compared to the father) falls far below the line of acceptability; for, as Woody recognizes, custody is customarily given to the mother (42). In any event, these findings take on importance only in the contested cases. In the cases where the parents agree, the relevance of the findings vary, depending on the judge's interest or concern in a particular case.

Should the mental health professional offer an opinion on the ultimate issue to be decided? Some say that the expert should not specifically name the best parent for the child. According to this view, the expert should limit his testimony to pointing out the individual's adequacies or inadequacies as a parent. The court, however, usually expects the expert in these cases to express an opinion on the ultimate issue. Justice Stewart of the United States Supreme Court recently observed that issues involving the family are the most difficult that courts have to face (43). Judge Botein of New York once commented, "A judge agonizes more about reaching the right result in a contested custody issue than about any other type decision he renders" (44).

Many observers say that the trial judge, however he may agonize, accepts the expert's opinion only when it is in accord with his personal assessment of the parties. After all, what judge does not feel that he knows more about parenting than any expert? The courts usually conclude that the balance is even, not wanting to impugn one parent, and then say that they rely on the testimony of the behavioral science expert to determine that the children are of such age that their needs are best met by the parent given custody. In any event, the expert's testimony makes it possible to pass the buck.

When all is said and done, it is really not clear how the decision-making responsibility is in fact shared, if at all, by the trial judge with the professionals who participate in the process (45). The experts do not vote or have a veto in the decision-making. However, it might be said that the use of expert testimony is frequently necessary to appease the parties—it, at least, makes them think they have gotten their money's worth.

In rendering an opinion that one party is more entitled than the other to be named custodian, it is incumbent upon the expert to interview both parties. Otherwise, the expert will be questioned on cross-examination: "Do you feel under the circumstances—not having seen the child or having seen the mother with the child or the father with the child—that you can make an assessment as to what would be in the best interests of the child?" (As the report is seen by the parties, the expert would be well-advised not to say that the mother looks older than her stated age.)

Proponents of psychological standards have acknowledged how problematic it is to evaluate relationships from a psychological perspective unless a highly trained person spends considerable time observing the interactions between the parent and child (46). Selma Fraiberg, an authority on child-rearing, reports that in many of the records she has examined, the professional staff attached to the court dispenses shabby counsel in which, she says, psychological ignorance and confusion are cloaked in pretentious scientific language (47). In a majority of our courts, she claims, the supporting staff, social workers and psychologists have neither the specialized professional training nor the vocational commitment to children which qualifies them as advisers to the court. Her conclusion is that these reports are worse than nothing. It is to be noted that the reports examined by Fraiberg were in Michigan, a state highly regarded for the caliber of its professional services. One supposes that the reports were probably more significant in settling disputes prior to hearing than they were at hearing.

Some may say that the best source of information lies with the treating mental health professional, should one be in the picture. The court or a contesting party might attempt to call upon the mental health professional, who may have seen either one of the parties or the child in the course of counseling or therapy either before or during the course of the divorce. Very often the court itself refers an individual for treatment in these cases. Questions of confidentiality are thus raised. On the one hand, it is argued that a court needs the information to make an informed judgment, while on the other hand, it is urged that a therapeutic relationship is impossible, if a client fears that what is communicated is subject to being divulged. There may be times when a party may wish his therapist to testify on his behalf, but that would be a private matter between them. The controversial issue arises when the court or a party calls on the counselor or therapist as a witness or deponent.

Various states have adopted one or more testimonial privileges allowing a party in certain professional relationships to refuse to disclose confidential communications, should they be demanded to do so in any legal proceeding. These privileges clearly do not apply when the court orders a party to submit to an examination, for, in such case, a true doctor-patient or other treatment relationship does not exist. For the counseling or treating relationship, Michigan has adopted a host of privileges for professionals, including: school officials (48), social workers (49), marriage counselors (50), psychologists (51), psychiatrists (52), and physicians (53), but apparently participation in a custody contest constitutes a waiver of these privileges. Curiously, of all the Michigan privileges, only the one on marriage counseling provides that "this privilege is not subject to waiver" (except where the counselor is a party defendant to a civil, criminal or disciplinary action arising from such counseling in which case the waiver is limited to that action) (54).

Though there is some variation in rulings among trial judges, the appellate court decisions around the country generally seem to hold that the "best interests of the child" outweigh the privilege of not releasing confidential information. Psychiatric history is relevant to the determination of "best interest," because character or mental and physical health of the parties is at issue in child custody disputes (55). Thus, in one Michigan case, the hospital record of the husband was admitted in a child custody contest indicating that he had once attempted suicide by drinking a toilet bowl cleaner (56). Moreover, the courts generally hold that the interests of young children outweigh the policies of confidentiality of alcohol and drug abuse patient records and the physician-patient relationship, and that production of the records, together with testimony of the patient's treatment center counselor, may be required (57). Under child abuse reporting statutes, there is a duty to come forward and report evidence of child abuse (58). Thus, in child custody litigation, as in other areas of the law involving children, the traditional privileges are waived to effect what is best for the child.

CONCLUSION

The general standard in child custody cases has shifted from parental-right to best interests of the child, but there is now a tendency to enact legislation that would set out presumptions limiting the discretion of the judge making a custody decision.

There are statutory presumptions that favor the parent over a nonparent, that give a preference to the wishes of a child over the age of 12 or 14, and that will favor joint custody if the proposals in a number of states pass. Under the law of evidence, overcoming a presumption requires persuasive evidence, which may not be available considering that experts are available to testify on opposite sides (59). Yet all of this may be more form than substance. Though not expressed in legislation, preference in fact is given to maternal custody of young children. Maternal love is, in fact, the decisional assumption, though there is much publicity to the contrary, encouraging litigation.

Since the mother will usually be awarded custody regardless of the statutory standard, and since it seems wise to discourage traumatic custody disputes whenever it is possible to do so, one might consider: should legislation be enacted establishing a presumption that the mother is entitled to custody of young children in order to discourage those husbands who might wish to contest? That is the recommendation of a number of commentators. Professor Areen observes: "The presumption resolves several value conflicts: it may well be true that because of the presumption some fathers who would be better custodians than their wives will either fail to seek custody or will be denied custody following a contest, but that disadvantage has a lower 'social cost' than the disadvantages of any alternative statutory formulation—more contested cases (with the trauma that contests seem to produce), more risk of a custody award to a father who will be only marginally better than the mother or even much worse" (60).

But with a maternal-preference presumption, what actions would be left to a father who wanted to counter a property demand? In any event, maternal preference must remain submerged as the decisional assumption. It would be sexist to say that women are necessarily best at nurturing (61). The true issue, however, is not whether paternal custody is in the best interest of the child. Ted of *Kramer v. Kramer* demonstrated that a father can make a good parent, but the demands of parenting cost Ted his job. The issue is really whether the country can tolerate absenteeism on the part of both sexes at a time when productivity is already low.

REFERENCES

1. Hamilton, W. (cartoon): *The New Yorker,* May 5, 1977, p. 84.
2. See, for example, Sterling Hayden's tale in his autobiography, *Wanderer.* New York: Avon, 1977.
3. 240 N.Y. 429, 148 N.E. 624.
4. Uniform Marriage and Divorce Act § 402, Comment to the section.
5. Casale v. Casale, 549 S.W.2d 805 (Ky. 1977), discussed in Comment, Paternal Custody of the Young Child under the Kentucky No-Fault Divorce, *Ky. L.J.,* 66:165, 1977.
6. Wallerstein, J. S. and Kelly, J. B.: *Surviving the Break-up: How Children Actually Cope with Divorce,* New York: Basic Books, 1980; Gardner, G.: Separation of the Parents and the Emotional Life of the Child, *Mental Hygiene* 40:53, 1956; Tuckman, J. and Regan, R. A.: Intactness of the Home and Behavioral Problems in Children, *J. Child Psychology & Psychiatry,* 7:225, 1966. But see M. Miller (ltr.), Divorce Impact on Children, *Psychology Today,* Jan. 1980, p. 5.
7. Hansen, R. W.: The Role and Rights of Children in Divorce Actions. *J. Family Law,* 6:1, 1966.
8. Uniform Marriage and Divorce Act § 301.
9. Mlyniec, W. J.: The Child Advocate in Private Custoday Disputes: A Role in Search of a Standard. *J. Family Law* 16:1, 1977.
10. Note, Alternatives to "Parental Rights" in Child Custody Disputes Involving Third Parties. *Yale L.J.,* 73:151 at 157, 1963.
11. P. 162.
12. P. 160.
13. P. 162.
14. Goldstein, J.: Psychoanalysis and Jurisprudence. *Yale L.J.,* 77:1053 at 1076, 1968.
15. Goldstein, J., Freud, A., and Solnit, A. J.: *Beyond the Best Interests of the Child.* New York: Free Press, 1973, p. 99.
16. P. 98.
17. Watson, A. S.: Family Law and Its Challenge for Psychiatry. *J. Family Law,* 2:71, 1962. The Children of Armageddon, Problems of Custody Following Divorce, *Syracuse L. Rev.,* 21:55, 1969.
18. Painter v. Bannister, 258 Iowa 1390, 140 N.W.2d 152 (1966).
19. March 21, 1967, published in *Newsletter,* American Orthopsychiatric Association, May 1968, p. 8. The resolution was approved by a mail vote of the membership of 517 yes to 17 no, or 97 percent approval.
20. In Stamper v. Stamper, Fam. L. Rep. 3:2541 (Wayne Cy. Circuit Ct., Mich, 1977), the court was faced with a practicing lesbian mother, who flaunted her lover, and an incapable, indecisive "workaholic." The court ordered joint custody to the father and mother.

21. Mnookin, J.: Child Custody Adjudication: Judicial Functions in the Face of Indeterminacy. *Law & Contemp. Prob.*, 39:226, 1975.
22. Okpaku, S. R.: Psychology: Impediment or Aid in Child Custody Cases? *Rutgers L. Rev.*, 29:1116 at 1152, 1976.
23. Areen, J.: *Cases and Materials on Family Law.* Mineola, N.Y.: Foundation Press, 1978, chap, 5, pp. 511-629.
24. Winnicott, D. W.: *The Child and the Family.* London: Tavistock, 1957.
25. Leavell, C.: Custody Disputes and the Proposed Model. *Georgia L. Rev.*, 2:162, 1968. The law specifically permits a judge to utilize "community resources in behavioral sciences" in determining a custody matter (MCLA § 722.27 (d)), but the decision to use such information is a matter of trial court discretion. *Siwik v. Siwik,* 280 N.W.2d 610 (Mich. App. 1979). Kentucky's statute provides: "The court may seek the advice of professional personnel, whether or not employed by the court on a regular basis. The advice given shall be in writing and made available by the court to counsel upon request. Counsel may examine as a witness any professional personnel consulted by the court." Ky. Rev. Stat. 403.290 (1972).
26. Rawls, J.: *A Theory of Justice.* Cambridge: Harvard University Press, 1971, p. 237.
27. Foster, H. and Freed, D.: Child Custody. *N.Y.U. L. Rev.*, 39:423, 1974.
28. Ellesworth, P. C. and Levy, R. J.: Legislative Reform of Child Custody Adjudication. *Law & Soc. Rev.*, 4:167 at 220, 1969.
29. Uniform Marriage and Divorce Act, § 402.
30. MCLA § 722.23. The criteria of the Michigan statute have been enacted in such states as Colorado, Florida, Indiana, Kentucky, Wisconsin, Texas and Oregon. D. Freed and H. Foster, Family Law in the Fifty States: An Overview. *Fam. L. Rep.*, 3:4047, 1977.
31. At least 20 states have statutes that specifically call for consideration of the child's wishes. Siegel, D. M. and Hurley, S.: The Role of the Child's Preference in Custody Proceedings. *Family L. Q.*, 11:1, 1977. Some of these statutes provide that the preference of children of age 12 or 14 or older is dispositive, unless the chosen parent is determined not to be a fit and proper person to have custody. Ga. Code Ann. § 30-127 (1977); Ohio Rev. Code Ann. § 3109.04 (1975); Tex. Fam. Code Ann. tit. 2, § 14.07 (1976). This legislation applies not only to original custody determinations incident to a divorce proceeding, but also to change of custody. Peacock v. Adams, 230 Ga. 774, 199 S.E. 2d 254 (Ga. 1973).
32. MCLA § 722.25.
33. Effectively, P.A. 1970 No. 91 repealed the "tender years" presumption. MCLA 722.541. Other states too have provided by legislation that there shall be no presumption that children of tender years, all other things being equal, should be given into the custody of their mother. Thus, legislation in New York provides: "In all cases there shall be no prima facie right to the custody of the child in either parent, but the court shall determine solely what is for the best interest of the child, and what will best promote its welfare and happiness." N.Y. Domestic Relations Law, sec. 240. Among the minority of cases awarding custody

to the father is Eigner v. Eigner, 79 Mich. App. 189, 261 N.W. 2d 254 (1977). In this case the court said that the mother's career and the fact that the children were looked after by a babysitter, along with the children's preference, warranted award of custody to the father, who lived on a farm. See also Gulyas v. Gulyas, 75 Mich. App. 138, 254 N.W. 2d 818 (1977), where the fact that the mother was an ambitious career woman and the father more a "homebody" warranted custody to the father.

34. Levy v. Levy, Supreme Court of New York, 1976, reported in *N.Y. Law Journal*, Jan. 29, 1976, p. 11. Apparently because of the criticisms or uncertainty about joint custody, a number of legislatures have been moved to enact a rule providing, in effect, that an award of joint custody is not incompatible with the best interests of the child. North Carolina has legislation authorizing joint custody "if clearly in the best interests of the child." N.C. Gen Stat. § 50-13.2 (b) (supp. vol. 2a 1975). Iowa's statute provides for joint custody where "justified." Iowa Code Ann. § 598.21 (supp. 1978-79). Wisconsin's statute provides where "the parties so agree and if the court finds that a joint custody arrangement would be in the best interests of the child or children." Wis. Stat. Ann. § 247.24 (1) (b) (cum. supp. 1978-79). Oregon's new statute authorizes the court to award custody to one party or jointly "as it may deem just and proper." Ore. Rev. Stat. § 107.105.

35. Michigan Senate Bill 254 of 1979 would amend the state's child custody act to establish a presumption that, in custody disputes between parents, "the best interest of the child is served by awarding joint custody or equal custody to the parents, unless the contrary is established by clear and convincing evidence." The Bill mandates that joint or equal custody *is* in the best interest of the child, prior to the court's analysis of the factors listed in the state's child custody act. The bill has not been adopted. See also H. Foster and D. Freed, Joint Custody: A Viable Alternative? *Trial*, 15:26, May 1979; J. B. Greif, Joint Custody: A Sociological Study, *Trial*, 15:32, May 1979; P. H. Nielson, Joint Custody: An Alternative for Divorced Parents, *UCLA L. Rev.*, 26:1084, 1979.

36. Wisconsin's statute defines "joint custody" as meaning that "both parties have equal rights and responsibilities to the minor child and neither parties' rights are superior." Wis. Stat. Ann. § 247.24 (1) (b) (supp. 1978-79). Michigan's proposed Senate Bill 254 of 1979 defines "equal custody" as providing each parent "with the physical presence of the child for the same amount of time" until the child reaches majority; and further, defines "joint custody" as permitting each parent "to concur in each decision which affects the overall welfare or development of a child and each decision which could have a lifetime impact upon the child."

37. Goldstein, J., Freud, A., and Solnit, A. J.: *Before the Best Interests of the Child*. New York: Free Press, 1979. Goldstein, J.: Psychoanalysis and a Jurisprudence of Child Placement—with Special Emphasis on the Role of Legal Counsel for Children, in D. N. Weisstaub (Ed.), *Law and Psychiatry II*. New York: Pergamon, 1979, p. 1.

38. Barnes v. Barnes, 77 Mich. App. 112, 258 N.W. 2d 65 (1977); Lewis v.

188 *Law and Ethics in the Practice of Psychiatry*

Lewis, 73 Mich. App. 563, 252 N.W. 2d 237 (1977); In re Custody of James B, 66 Mich. App. 133, 238 N.W. 2d 419 (1975); Zawisa v. Zawisa, 61 Mich. App. 1, 232 N.W. 2d 275 (1975); Hilbert v. Hilbert, 57 Mich. App. 247, 225 N.W. 2d 697 (1974).

39. Hunter, N. D. and Polikoff, N. D.: Custody Rights of Lesbian Mothers: Legal Theory and Litigation Strategy. *Buffalo L. Rev.*, 25:691, 1976.
40. Leonard, M. J.: Fathers and Daughters: The Significance of "Fathering" in the Psychosexual Development of the Girl. *Int. J. Psa.*, 47:325, 1966.
41. Woody, R. H.: *Getting Custody/Winning the Last Battle of the Marital War.* New York: Macmillan, 1978.
42. P. 57. And custody was awarded to the mother in the prize-winning and tear-jerking film "Kramer vs. Kramer" (based on Avery Corman's novel) even though the mother had abandoned the child. In this story, the wife walked out on her husband and six-year-old son "to find herself," only to return 18 months later to fight for the custody of the child. Said the court: "The court is guided by the best interests of the child and rules the best interests of this child, who is of tender age, will be served by his return to the mother." Corman, A.: *Kramer versus Kramer.* New York: Random House, 1977, p. 233.

Carol Lowery, psychologist at the University of Kentucky, surveyed judges in that state for their assessment of the main factors, and she came up with the following items in this rank order: 1) mental stability of each parent; 2) each parent's sense of responsibility to the child; 3) biological relationship to the child (when one parent is a stepparent); 4) each parent's moral character; 5) each parent's ability to provide stable involvement in a community; 6) each parent's affection for the child; 7) keeping the child with siblings; 8) each parent's ability to provide access to schools; 9) keeping a young child with the mother; 10) physical health of each parent; 11) the wishes of the parents; 12) professional advice; 13) biological relationship to the child (when one parent is an adoptive parent); 14) each parent's financial sufficiency; 15) the child's wishes; 16) length of time each parent has had custody; 17) each parent's ability to provide contact with the child's other relatives; 18) each parent's ability to provide access to other children of about the same age; 19) each parent's ability or intention to provide a two-parent home; and 20) placing a child with the parent of the same sex. The ranking of maternal preference in ninth place was surprising. Lowery wondered whether the judges were being less than honest in their ranking. Lowery, C. R.: Child Custody Decisions in Divorce Proceedings: A Survey of Judges, paper presented at the Biennial Meeting of the American Psychology-Law Society, on Oct 19, 1979, in Baltimore, Md.
43. Parham v. J.R., 99 S. Ct. 2493 at 2515, 1979.
44. *Trial Judge*, 1952, p. 273.
45. Mnookin, R. H., *op. cit. supra* note 21.
46. Cited in R. H. Mnookin, *op. cit. supra* note 21.
47. Fraiberg, S.: *Every Child's Birthright: In Defense of Mothering.* New York: Basic Books, 1977, p. 88.

48. MCLA § 600.2165.
49. MCLA § 400.35, 338.1764.
50. MCLA § 338.1043.
51. MCLA §338.1018.
52. MCLA § 600.2157.
53. MCLA § 600.2157.
54. MCLA § 338.1043.
55. Allen v. Dept. of Human Resources, 540 S.W. 2d 597 (Ky. 1976).
56. Feldman v. Feldman, 55 Mich. App. 147, 222 N.W. 2d 2 (1974). But in the case of In re "B", Appeal of Dr. Loren Roth, 394 A.2d 419 (Pa. 1978), involving a juvenile placement proceeding, Justice Manderino of the Pennsylvania Supreme Court said that a patient's constitutional right of privacy protects the confidentiality of communications in psychotherapy. In this case, the caseworker assigned to aid the court had found out about the mother's psychiatric treatment while doing a background investigation, and had recommended getting the record. The juvenile court's psychiatrist also recommended getting the mother's record, but one may ask whether there was really any need for it in order to determine the disposition of her son (who had been adjudicated a delinquent after participating in four auto thefts). Indeed, Justice Roberts in a concurring opinion concluded that the mother's psychiatric record was not needed and hence he would not engage in any discussion of constitutional questions. 394 A.2d at 426.
57. Matter of Doe Children, 93 Misc. 2d 479, 402 N.Y.S. 2d 958 (1978). In federally-supported alcohol and drug treatment programs, confidentiality of records is a legal requirement except as defined in the exclusions cited in the regulation. No records of identity, diagnosis, prognosis, or treatment mentioned in connection with any drug-abuse prevention may be used to conduct any investigation of the patient or to initiate or substantiate any criminal charges against the patient. Confidentiality of Alcohol and Drug Abuse Patient Records, Federal Register DHEW-PHS, vol. 40 (127), July 1976.
58. The statutory obligation to report suspected child abuse to state authorities takes priority over confidentiality guarantees. The 1975 Michigan Child Protection Law specifically states that privileged or confidential communication is "abrogated" in order for treatment personnel to report child abuse cases or to present information in a child abuse court case. The only exception under this law is confidential communication between lawyer and client. Under the Michigan law, confidentiality is also waived in order for the state Child Protective Services (which has responsibility for the child protection in Michigan) to gain information and assistance from other agencies and professionals in child abuse cases.
59. Bahr v. Bahr, 60 Mich. App. 354, 230 N.W. 2d 430 (1975).
60. J. Areen, *op. cit. supra* note 23, at p. 541.
61. Roth, A.: The Tender Years Presumption in Child Custody Disputes. *J. Family Law*, 15:423, 1977.

8

Mock - Trial Demonstration

Judge: Carol Haberman, LL.B.
Plaintiff Attorney: Carol Tucker, LL.B.
Defense Attorney: John Specia, LL.B.
Plaintiff Psychiatrist: Jonas Rappeport, M.D.
Defense Psychiatrist: Elissa Benedek, M.D.

Editor's note: What follows is the minimally edited transcript of a mock-trial, presented live and unrehearsed at the American College of Psychiatrists' meeting. Aside from Dr. Rada's introductory remarks and certain omissions noted by Judge Haberman, the material very closely approaches that which might be offered at an actual hearing.

Dr. Rada: I should like, first of all, to introduce Judge Carol Haberman. Judge Haberman is the Judge of the 45th District Court in San Antonio. Our expert attorneys are Carol Tucker and John Specia. Ms. Tucker took an M.S.W. degree before going to law school, and she is now an attorney in private practice. Mr. Specia is an attorney for the Department of

190

Human Resources and a child welfare attorney. Dr. Jonas Rappeport, Chief Medical Officer of the Supreme Bench of Baltimore, is going to be one of the expert witnesses. Dr. Elissa Benedek, the other expert witness, is Director of Training and Education at the Center for Forensic Psychiatry, Ann Arbor, and Clinical Professor of Psychiatry at the University of Michigan. John Specia will serve as the plaintiff's attorney and Carol Tucker will serve as the defense attorney, so Carol will be giving direct examination to Elissa and John will be giving direct examination to Jonas.

This is a child custody final hearing, and it is important to know the setting. There have been many previous witnesses, so we are getting into the middle of a trial where many of the facts have already been established.

It is also important to know that there has been a planned lack of precision, which the attorneys are finding difficult to handle at this point. The reason is that we wanted to promote the kind of atmosphere which would allow for some mistakes. In order to assure this, we have even primed one of the witnesses, who is going to have to present testimony contrary to the manner in which he might normally do.

Finally, the expert witnesses have been qualified before the curtain rises. We'll start with Judge Haberman, who will read to you the basic facts of the case as they currently stand, and then we'll call the expert witnesses.

Judge Haberman: Thank you. Ladies and gentlemen, today we have Joan and John Smith before us. Joan and John were separated two years ago following a marriage of 12 years. The separation was an emotional, trying, and unpleasant experience for both parties. They both have many unresolved feelings regarding the reasons for the divorce and the divorce itself. The Smiths have three children: a son, John, Jr., age 14; a daughter, Ann, age 10; and a son, Calvin, age six. Mr. Smith is petitioning at this time, which is the final hearing, for full custody of the children. This action was prompted by his oldest son's indicating to him that he did not want to live with his mother and by stories that he had heard from the son and others that his ex-wife had developed a severe drinking problem which affected her ability to care for the children.

These are additional facts. Joan Smith is a 31-year-old white woman who married her former husband when age 17. She was several months pregnant at the time of the marriage. She has a high-school education, and is planning on returning to college. She is a dramatic and histrionic person, with a history of multiple somatic conditions and complaints over the years and a series of hospitalizations and operations for which no organic cause was found. She has had two hospitalizations for severe depression, each following the birth of a child. The second hospitalization was prompted by suicidal and infanticidal fears. She has been accused of having a severe drinking problem, but she is interested in the arts and is a frequent, though not a consistent, churchgoer.

The father is a 33-year-old accountant, described as an obsessive-compulsive personality with a strong, authoritarian manner. He is a strict disciplinarian, nonimaginative and not demonstratively affectionate. He has a bad temper and has been accused of hitting his wife on several occasions. At this time, I will call on the plaintiff's attorney to present the first expert witness for this phase. Mr. John Specia.

Mr. Specia: Your Honor, I would like to call Dr. Jonas Rappeport, please.

Judge Haberman: Dr. Rappeport, you may come right up here, sir. Dr. Rappeport, do you swear to tell the truth, the whole truth, and nothing but the truth in the testimony you are about to offer, so help you, God?

Dr. Rappeport: I do.

Judge Haberman: You may be seated.

Mr. Specia: Doctor, for the record, would you state your name?

Dr. Rappeport: Dr. Jonas Rappeport.

Mr. Specia: And what is your present position?

Dr. Rappeport: I am a psychiatrist. I function as the Chief Medical Officer for the Supreme Bench of Baltimore.

Mr. Specia: Your Honor, with the Court's permission, we would like to stipulate as to the expert status of this witness.

Judge Haberman: Is there an objection?

Ms. Tucker: No objection.

Judge Haberman: The Court will receive it as stipulated.

Mr. Specia: Have you examined Mr. Smith?

Dr. Rappeport: Yes, I have, sir.

Mr. Specia: And who requested this examination?

Dr. Rappeport: You did, sir.

Mr. Specia: Has Mr. Smith authorized you to testify at this hearing?

Dr. Rappeport: Yes, he has, sir.

Mr. Specia: Are you being compensated for your testimony?

Dr. Rappeport: Yes, indeed!

(*laughter in the courtroom*)

Mr. Specia: Are you receiving your normal compensation?

Dr. Rappeport: I am receiving my normal and customary fee for the amount of time I have devoted to this case.

Mr. Specia: What type of evaluation did you conduct on Mr. Smith?

Dr. Rappeport: I interviewed Mr. Smith on Tuesday, February 5 for approximately one and one-half hours.

Mr. Specia: Is this type of examination sufficient for you to draw some conclusions?

Dr. Rappeport: I believe that the information that I obtained from Mr. Smith as a result of my examination was sufficient and adequate for me to form an opinion; yes sir.

Mr. Specia: What is your general impression of Mr. Smith?

Dr. Rappeport: My general impression of Mr. Smith is that he is a very competent individual, albeit somewhat rigid; one we might call an obsessive-compulsive personality, which is a quality which serves a useful purpose in his career. He is a certified public accountant, and I might say that obsessive-compulsive accountants are the best kind. (*laughter in the courtroom*) I believe that he has a very strong interest in his children and is concerned about their care and nurturance and would like to do the very best he can to help them grow up and to be responsible citizens.

Mr. Specia: For my benefit, are there any problems with being a parent and being an obsessive-compulsive personality?

Dr. Rappeport: Problems with being an obsessive-compulsive personality in terms of parenting? I think that depends on the degree, but, generally speaking, people with this personality structure are seen in the professions, law, medicine, accountancy, other fields. These are people who tend to be somewhat precise, exact, authoritarian, demanding of themselves, and sometimes demanding of others. They like a well-structured and organized life. On the negative side, they may have some difficulty in expressing emotion in any direct and clear manner. Instead, they tend to keep themselves well-controlled, but, in terms of helping children grow and develop, they certainly do offer structure and organization, scheduling, and so on, to their lives.

Mr. Specia: What is Mr. Smith's concern, concerning the children and the care they are receiving from their mother?

Dr. Rappeport: Well, Mr. Smith tells me that his basic concern is that his wife is unstable. He left her because of the numerous fights they had over her housekeeping. She was nowhere near as good a housekeeper and mother as his mother had been. His father was a policeman for the city police force, who worked the evening shift from four to 12 p.m., but he did get to see his father in the summer when he helped him on his other law-maintenance job, although not a whole lot during the winter. Mother was a very exact, careful, churchgoing housekeeper and Mr. Smith's wife, Mrs. Smith, did not meet those qualifications. Further, the children have reported to him, particularly the oldest boy, that she has been drinking excessively, and Mr. Smith, himself, believes on a few occasions when he visited the house that she was intoxicated. He was quite upset by the fact that she is apparently dating, and he believes has been involved with other men in the house when the children have been around.

Mr. Specia: Doctor, let's discuss that a little bit. What would be the effect on the two younger children, particularly Ann and Calvin, of their mother fooling around, as you said, with other men in their presence, prior to the divorce?

Dr. Rappeport: I would say, generally speaking, this would not be very helpful, particularly for a six- and a 10-year-old child to be exposed to what might be considered infidelity or overt sexual behavior with a person other than their father. I think this might well interfere with the children's psychosexual development, cause them, perhaps, some overstimulation, creating anxiety and tension in their lives and, at the very least, confusion as to the role of fidelity in behavior.

Mr. Specia: What would this tell you about the judgment of Mrs. Smith?

Dr. Rappeport: This would indicate to me that Mrs. Smith is somewhat impulsive, and that she seems to be unable to delay her needs for a more appropriate time or occasion, and that her judgment is not good. I would question her devotion to the care of her children.

Mr. Specia: You are aware of the fact that John, Jr., age 14, has requested that he live with his father?

Dr. Rappeport: That is correct, sir.

Mr. Specia: What do you see as the significance of this?

Dr. Rappeport: Well, I think this might indicate his desire to have a closer relationship and a better identification with his father. It indicates an existing identification with his father, which is certainly a healthy model in a 14-year-old. It may indicate, on the other hand, a negative identification with his mother. It depends on how one looks at it. The average 14-year-old is beginning to get into a phase of his life when he doesn't care too much for his father and might wonder how his father got to be so stupid in 33 years. But this kid, I think, is being torn in his situation, and feels dissatisfied with his life with his mother, and wants to be with father.

Mr. Specia: What are the needs of a 14-year-old boy in a home?

Dr. Rappeport: I would think a 14-year-old boy needs some structure, some opportunity for a regular organized schedule, since at this time he is struggling with his own sexual development, his identity, his reemergence of what we call his infantile fantasies. He needs to deal with these problems. A relationship with a seductive or sometimes intoxicated mother could cause severe problems for him, as he is trying to learn how to integrate and control his own sexual development.

Mr. Specia: What are the basic needs of the other Smith children? I know you didn't get to see Ann or Calvin, but what are the needs of a 10-year-old girl and a six-year-old boy in their home in order to develop into healthy human beings?

Dr. Rappeport: Being a good obsessive-compulsive, myself, I favor some structure and security. I think the most important thing all children need is an integrated family and security. Unfortunately, these children have a split family, so that that part of the situation we have to take as we find it. But, I do think they need security, regular scheduling, some recognition that somebody who is a caring person will be there when they need them and will not be functioning in an erratic fashion. It wouldn't even have to be mother or father, as long as it's somebody with whom they feel comfortable and secure. The 10-year-old girl certainly should have, if possible, a good mother-model from which to establish her as a role model. And, as Mr. Smith described Mrs. Smith, she didn't quite fit that description by most people's standards.

Mr. Specia: Doctor, assume that Mrs. Smith has a serious drinking problem. What type of impact would a mother with a serious drinking problem have, if she were the sole caretaker, or primary caretaker?

Dr. Rappeport: I would think, at the very least, the result for the children would be insecurity from an individual who cannot control herself and maintain any consistency. It depends, of course, on what her behavior is when she's intoxicated. Certainly slovenliness, or passing out, would not be what most of us would accept as a good model for a child.

Mr. Specia: Assume further that Mrs. Smith has expressed somatic complaints, spends much time in bed, and has had prior hospitalizations where there was no observable reason for these hospitalizations. How would this type of conduct affect the children?

Dr. Rappeport: I would think it would further reduce their security. Their mother, the one they depend on, is in bed half the time or drunk half the time. This would certainly have them frightened and worried as to who's going to take care of them. What's the situation going to be when they arise in the morning or when they get home in the evening?

Mr. Specia: Did Mr. Smith talk to you about his plans for caring for the children while he's at work?

Dr. Rappeport: Yes. Mr. Smith said that he would be home at six o'clock every evening except for the three months prior to the tax season, when, of course, he is busy with income tax preparation. He would try to be with them on weekends except that he also does a little side-job as a special tax consultant for corporations on Saturdays and Sundays. However, he would move in with his parents—his mother is 63 years old—and he would hire a maid in order to help his mother give the kids some care. He is active in the Kiwanis Club and some other groups, so that he goes to a lot of night meetings. Despite his desire, his professional requirements are such, and also his personal requirements, I guess, that he would not be home too much, except that he would provide the security of his parents' home.

Mr. Specia: How would Mr. Smith serve as a role model for these children? He seems to be a civic-minded, hard-working individual.

Dr. Rappeport: Well, I think he represents an upstanding—as you said, civic-minded—involved, well-controlled individual.

(laughter in courtroom)

Judge Haberman: Order in the Court.

Mr. Specia: If you had to pick between a home that was chaotic, where there was no consistency of care, the mother had many problems, there were frequent male visitors, and a home that was stable, what would you pick as being the preferable type of home?

(laughter in courtroom)

Dr. Rappeport: I would certainly pick the least detrimental alternative, which I would see as the more firm, stable environment.

Mr. Specia: Doctor, in your professional opinion, do you believe that John Smith has the requisite ability to provide a safe, loving, and secure home for these children?

Dr. Rappeport: Yes sir, I do.

Mr. Specia: I'll pass the witness.

Judge Haberman: You may proceed with cross-examination at this time.

Ms. Tucker: Thank you, Your Honor. Dr. Rappeport, you've described Mr. Smith as rigid, is that correct? And as authoritarian?

Dr. Rappeport: Yes, ma'am.

Ms. Tucker: Right. Would you say he's a driving sort of person?

Dr. Rappeport: Driving?

Ms. Tucker: Drives himself, others?

Dr. Rappeport: Yes, I would say that he's a driving sort of person.

Ms. Tucker: Isn't it true that kids need hugs, too?

Dr. Rappeport: Oh, yes!

Ms. Tucker: And can you see Mr. Smith giving that kind of support to children?

Dr. Rappeport: I think he would try to. I don't think it would be easy for him to do a whole lot of it. He might be helped; he might be helped with some counseling to learn—or to even pretend, which isn't as good as giving it honestly— (*laughter in courtroom*) to give more affection.

Judge Haberman: Order in the Court!

Ms. Tucker: Are you advocating pretend hugs, then?

Dr. Rappeport: They are better than none. (*laughter in courtroom*)

Ms. Tucker: That's true, but if you had a choice of hugs, a real hug or a pretend hug, which one would be best for the child?

Dr. Rappeport: Certainly, real affection is better than pretended affection.

Ms. Tucker: Now we hear that Mr. Smith has very high expectations of the children. Does that make sense with what you know of Mr. Smith?

Dr. Rappeport: Yes, it does.

Ms. Tucker: What about this quizzing with homework? We also hear that he sort of gives them the third degree. Does that make sense from what you know of Mr. Smith?

Dr. Rappeport: I think that fits in with Mr. Smith; that he's very interested and desirous of knowing: 1) what his children are learning, and 2) what his wife isn't giving them.

Ms. Tucker: Dr. Rappeport, what causes a peptic ulcer? What kind of person gets a peptic ulcer?

Dr. Rappeport: Well, there are lots of arguments and theories, but in Mr. Smith's case, I suspect his peptic ulcer may well be related to his inability to express some of his feelings.

Ms. Tucker: And similarly, Doctor, what causes hypertension?

Dr. Rappeport: Similar dynamics may be involved.

Ms. Tucker: So, generally, would you agree with the statement that these symptoms are indicative of someone who is sitting on a lot of anger?

Dr. Rappeport: Yes.

Ms. Tucker: All right. And would you agree that Mr. Smith has difficulty in expressing warm feelings, tender feelings?

Dr. Rappeport: Yes.

Ms. Tucker: And would you agree that he has difficulty in expressing angry feelings, at least before he explodes?

Dr. Rappeport: I doubt if Mr. Smith ever explodes; his ulcer does. (*laughter*)

Ms. Tucker: Well, are you aware that in the past he has beaten Joan Smith, sitting next to me?

Dr. Rappeport: He told me he had hit his wife a few times.

Ms. Tucker: And are you aware that her drinking really started after the beatings? That she drank the most after she was beaten?

Dr. Rappeport: I'm not aware of that, no.

Ms. Tucker: All right. And speaking of Joan's drinking. Are you also aware that Joan, for the past three months, has been active in AA?

Dr. Rappeport: No, I wasn't.

Ms. Tucker: And are you aware that in the past three months, Joan has not had one drop of alcohol.

Dr. Rappeport: I think that is wonderful.

Ms. Tucker: Thank you, Doctor. Now that you have been made aware of the fact that Joan has been totally sober for the past three months, would this fact change your mind as to her ability to care for her three children?

Dr. Rappeport: Probably not.

Ms. Tucker: And why is that, Doctor?

Dr. Rappeport: If the date is three months, that's the date that the custody suit was initiated, and I suspect that, for whatever reasons and upon whoever's advice, she ran to AA pretty quick to try to do something about the problem. Three months of sobriety is very, very little in the life of an alcoholic.

Ms. Tucker: But somebody with motivation and somebody with a really deep problem would not be able to make it for three months, would they, Doctor?

Dr. Rappeport: I admire her intentions, but I'm not willing to accept that this represents any real change in her basic personality.

Ms. Tucker: Doctor, you are making a lot of assumptions today about Joan and about the children, and, in fact, you have seen only Mr. Smith; is that correct?

Dr. Rappeport: That's correct.

Ms. Tucker: So you, then, have no firsthand knowledge of anyone in this family other than Mr. Smith; is that not correct?

Dr. Rappeport: That's absolutely correct.

Ms. Tucker: And, in fact, you don't know if Mr. Smith was exaggerating in what he told you?

Dr. Rappeport: I don't *know*. My clinical impression was that he was being honest and straightforward and, based on my total picture of Mr. Smith, people like him find it difficult to exaggerate and certainly difficult to lie, so my impression was that he was a reliable historian.

Ms. Tucker: Would it not serve Mr. Smiths' purpose, in fact, to lie to you?

Dr. Rappeport: Yes.

Ms. Tucker: Dr. Rappeport, is it good professional practice for you to come into Court today having seen only Mr. Smith?

Dr. Rappeport: It is not.

(*laughter in courtroom*)

Ms. Tucker: Now, Doctor, we know that Mr. Smith is a CPA, right? And you've testified about his hours, that he will be working the three months during tax season, right? And you've also testified as to his moonlighting as a tax consultant and to his civic activities, correct?

Dr. Rappeport: Yes.

Ms. Tucker: So, then, isn't it true that the people who will be raising these children will be the paternal grandparents and not Mr. Smith?

Dr. Rappeport: To a large extent. Most of their time will be with the paternal grandparents.

Ms. Tucker: And you are advocating this over a warm, loving mother?

Dr. Rappeport: Mrs. Smith was not described to me as a warm, loving mother by Mr. Smith.

Ms. Tucker: And again, Doctor, we're going just on descriptions, isn't that true?

Dr. Rappeport: That's correct.

Ms. Tucker: And no firsthand knowledge?

Dr. Rappeport: No, ma'am.

Ms. Tucker: Thank you. I'll pass the witness.

Mr. Specia: Doctor, is there anything wrong with good grandparents?

Dr. Rappeport: Having good grandparents? No, it's very helpful.

Mr. Specia: Is it more important for children to be with their natural parents, whoever they are, or to be with consistent, loving people who are giving them care?

Dr. Rappeport: I think most evidence indicates that consistent, loving care is more important than blood bonds.

Mr. Specia: Did you get the impression of Mr. Smith's parents that they were people who could do this?

Dr. Rappeport: My general impression was that they were certainly consistent, conforming, religious, competent people, who seemed to have, as best I could tell from Mr. Smith in trying to evaluate him, some capacity for giving.

Mr. Specia: He has achieved many successes in his life, is that not true?

Dr. Rappeport: Yes.

Mr. Specia: Is it good to have expectations of children?

Dr. Rappeport: Oh, I think it not only is good, but if children are to succeed, they have to be expected to succeed.

Mr. Specia: Has Mr. Smith expressed a desire to work on being a loving, feeling parent?

Dr. Rappeport: I discussed this with Mr. Smith, and he expressed to me that he really wanted his children. It was clear that some of this was based on his true desire for his children as a father, his love, his blood ties, and so on. Some was probably based on his need to retaliate or get back at his wife. I discussed with him his difficulty in expressing feelings, the limited relationship he had with his father, and my suggestion was that, if he obtained custody of the children, he should seriously consider getting some help from one of the local social agencies in perhaps trying to learn how to better relate to the children and learn their needs as opposed to his ideas of their needs.

Mr. Specia: Did he indicate whether he would do this?

Dr. Rappeport: He expressed great willingness to do whatever was necessary to help his children.

Mr. Specia: Regarding his plan of care for the children, do you feel that it is adequate?

Dr. Rappeport: Yes, I do, sir.

Mr. Specia: Have you had any experience with problems of alcoholism?

Dr. Rappeport: Yes, I have, sir.

Mr. Specia: How much experience have you had with these problems?

Dr. Rappeport: At one time in my career, for approximately a year, I ran an alcoholic service in one of the state hospitals, and throughout my career from time to time I have treated and frequently evaluated and recommended treatment for alcoholics.

Mr. Specia: What type or rate of recidivism is normal in alcoholic treatment?

Dr. Rappeport: Well, I think the rate of recidivism is exceedingly high. I don't know a number, but the longer one is sober, the lower the recidivism. It's an inverse relationship.

Mr. Specia: Is it important to respect the wishes of a 14-year-old boy as to where he wants to live?

Dr. Rappeport: Generally so; although, as a psychiatrist, I would want to know where he's coming from and the reasons that he is expressing these wishes. If I can't find out, I think basically, at 14, one should consider accepting his wishes.

Mr. Specia: Considering the information that you've been provided by opposing counsel, have you changed your opinion as to whether or not Mr. Smith could be a good parent in this case?

Dr. Rappeport: No, sir, I have not.

Mr. Specia: Thank you. I pass the witness.

Judge Haberman: Any other questions of the witness?

Ms. Tucker: No, Your Honor.

Judge Haberman: At this time you may be excused, Doctor. Will either of you need Dr. Rappeport for further questioning at a later time?

Mr. Specia: No, Your Honor.

Judge Haberman: Then you may be excused to go back to work or wherever you please.

Ms. Tucker: Your Honor, at this time, we would like to call Dr. Benedek.

Judge Haberman [to the audience]: Just as an explanation, the plaintiff would normally be resting his case, and the defense attorney would normally present a number of witnesses, perhaps even prior to this primary witness, for this purpose. It could be a grandparent or someone else very close to the family that the party may wish to have on the stand prior to this witness. So please remember that the Court has already heard from perhaps two or three other witnesses before Dr. Benedek takes the stand.

[to Dr. Benedek] Raise your right hand and be sworn, please. Do you swear to tell the truth, the whole truth and nothing but the truth in the testimony you are about to offer, so help you God?

Dr. Benedek: I do.

Judge Haberman: Then you may be seated, and you may proceed, counsel.

Ms. Tucker: Would you please state your name for the record.

Dr. Benedek: Elissa P. Benedek, M.D.

Ms. Tucker: And what is your present position?

Dr. Benedek: I am a licensed physician in the state of Michigan and psychiatrist. I am Director of Research and Training at the Center for Forensic Psychiatry.

Ms. Tucker: Your Honor, in the interest of time, we will ask the Court to allow us to stipulate to Dr. Benedek's qualifications.

Judge Haberman: Is there any question on the stipulation from the counsel?

Mr. Specia: I have no objections, Your Honor.

Judge Haberman: Then the Court will receive the stipulations at this time.

Ms. Tucker: Doctor, have you had occasion to evaluate the entire Smith family?

Dr. Benedek: Yes, counsel, I have. I have evaluated Mrs. Smith, Mr. Smith, the three Smith children, and the maternal grandmother.

Ms. Tucker: Dr. Benedek, are you aware of the existence of a patient-therapist privilege in Texas?

Dr. Benedek: Yes I am.

Ms. Tucker: And has the privilege been raised and discussed with the family and waived by its members?

Dr. Benedek: Yes, with each of the members of the Smith family that I interviewed. I talked with them about the fact that I would need to submit a report to the Court, and I might possibly have to testify in court and that what they said to me would not be confidential. I assured myself that all the members, including the children, understood this and asked them to sign a statement which I had prepared. They did understand that there would be no confidentiality or privilege.

Ms. Tucker: Thank you, Doctor. Now, Doctor, what was the nature of your evaluation of Joan Smith?

Dr. Benedek: I did a complete psychiatric evaluation of Joan Smith. That included taking a history of the circumstances surrounding the divorce and her reasons for requesting child custody, a complete past history, medical history, history of her own development, including school, work history, history of alcohol and drug abuse. Finally, I did a mental status evaluation.

Ms. Tucker: Would you please describe Joan, briefly, in terms of her current functioning.

Dr. Benedek: Yes. Mrs. Smith is a 31-year-old woman, who is currently living at home with her three children and has the sole responsibility for care of her children. She is working as a secretary and intends to go back to college to complete her education. She spends a great deal of time with her children. After work, she is solely responsible for the care of her children. She plans activities for the children on weekends and follows through with these activities. She's responsible for the complete medical care of her children. One of the youngsters, Calvin, has a disorder, a psychiatric disorder. She has arranged for psychiatric care for Calvin, and sees that Calvin makes his appointments. In addition, she has gone to Alcoholics Anonymous. She recognizes that, under stress, she tends to drink a great deal and has had contact in the past with Alcoholics Anonymous. During the time of the two psychiatric hospitalizations, she was introduced to that self-help group and found it helpful for her. Thus, recognizing that she would be under a great deal of stress at the time of this custody hearing, she herself decided that it might be sensible for her to find some support outside of her family, and she has gone to Alcoholics Anonymous.

Ms. Tucker: Have you formed, Doctor, an opinion as to Joan's overall emotional health at this point in time?

Dr. Benedek: Yes, counsel, I have.

Ms. Tucker: And what is that opinion?

Dr. Benedek: It is my opinion that, despite the fact that Mrs. Smith is mildly depressed, in some fashion reactive to the divorce proceedings and the child custody proceedings, she is generally functioning quite well.

Ms. Tucker: So you feel, then, that it's a sign of strength that she sought out AA?

Dr. Benedek: Yes, counsel, I do.

Ms. Tucker: And do you find that her motivation to keep her problem under control is genuine?

Dr. Benedek: Yes, counsel, I do believe it's genuine.

Ms. Tucker: And are you optimistic about her ability to do this, to keep it under control?

Dr. Benedek: Yes; Mrs. Smith has shown a great deal of care and concern and ability to plan for her future and for that of the children. She recognizes that she will be, as a single parent, under a great deal of stress, and it will be a difficult role for her to assume. She has experienced some difficulties in the past two years, but she sought appropriate help for herself and her child.

Ms. Tucker? What about Joan's mothering skills, her ability to care for the three children?

Dr. Benedek: Throughout the history of the marriage, Mrs. Smith has really had the primary responsibility for care of the children. That is to say, she has been with the children for the vast majority of the time; she has cared for them daily, looking after them when they have been ill, attending their school conferences, planning activities for them, spending time alone with them. She shows a great deal of care and concern for all three of her children and has demonstrated that care and concern throughout her years as a mother.

Ms. Tucker: Now, you also saw Mr. Smith?

Dr. Benedek: Yes, counsel, I did.

Ms. Tucker: And what kind of individual did you find him to be?

Dr. Benedek: Mr. Smith was a very rigid, controlled man who was unable to express any affection or warm feelings for his wife or for his children. He indicated that he felt that he had been mistreated by all of them. He had been a provider, had been the sole source of support for the family, and had never been truly appreciated. He indicated that he had not spent time with the children. . . .

Mr. Specia: Objection, Your Honor.

Judge Haberman: State the objection.

Mr. Specia: I'd like counsel to restrict herself to a question-and-answer format, please.

Judge Haberman: Sustained, counsel.

Ms. Tucker: Doctor, did you find Mr. Smith to be a warm person?

Dr. Benedek: No, counsel, I did not.

Ms. Tucker: Did you find him to have been involved with the day-to-day activities of his family?

Dr. Benedek: No. I questioned Mr. Smith in great detail to find out what, in fact, he had done with the children, and, in point of fact, he had, throughout his years as a father, spent very little time with the children. When the children were ill, he had his wife take them to the physician; when there were medical plans to be followed through, he never took any part in those plans. He never attended a school conference, despite the fact that the school, because of Calvin's difficulty, had specifically requested his presence at a conference. He was not involved in any activities with the children, and, in fact, could not describe anything that he had done with the youngsters prior to the last three months.

Ms. Tucker: Thank you, Doctor. Let's talk for a moment about John, Jr., whom you also saw. What was your opinion of the state of John, Jr.'s emotional health?

Dr. Benedek: John, Jr., as are all the children, is mildly depressed. John was quite able to talk about feeling sad about the breakup of the marriage. John indicated that he was very confused about which parent he wanted to live with. He had a great deal of concern about his father and had noticed his father crying recently, something he had never seen before.

He felt very worried about what would happen if he chose not to live with his father, and that is the reason, he explained to me, he had told people, including his father, that he would like to live with him. However, John said that he really wasn't sure about that, whether that was a legitimate reason for wanting to live with his father.

Ms. Tucker: Did it seem to you, Doctor, that John was perhaps trying to protect his father?

Dr. Benedek: Yes, counsel, it did.

Ms. Tucker: I see. Now, what about Ann? Ann is 10 years old, is that correct?

Dr. Benedek: Yes.

Ms. Tucker: And what kind of child is she, how well put together is she?

Dr. Benedek: Ann is a very lively, articulate youngster. We talked about the divorce. What did divorce mean? And what would it mean in terms of her future? We spent a great deal of time talking about Ann's relationship with her mother, the fact that she spent a great deal of time with her mother, that she enjoyed being with her mother, and that more recently, in the past three months, her father had begun to pay attention to her. Ann clearly expressed a preference for living with her mother and growing up and being like her mother.

Ms. Tucker: Did Ann appear at all frightened about the prospect of not living with her mother?

Dr. Benedek: We talked about the fact that, although I would make a recommendation, that it would be up to the Court to decide. Ann said that she was worried that if she did not live with her mother, her father would not allow her mother to visit, and she said that when her father loses his temper, he gets very mad. She said she has seen him hit her mother on occasion, and she was quite frightened that, if indeed she were to live with her father, and her mother asked to visit, her mother might be beaten by her father.

Ms. Tucker: Did Ann seem at all fearful of her own safety?

Dr. Benedek: Ann said that she was not concerned that her father would beat her. She's seen him get very angry and very explosive, and she described watching her father clench and unclench his fists. She's a very perceptive child, and she said that, at this point, she was not frightened of her father, but she was frightened about what her father might do to her mother.

Ms. Tucker: Did Ann make any comments to you as to the quality of mothering that she herself received from Joan?

Dr. Benedek: Ann talked about the fun she had with her mother, how she liked to go with her mother to the store and help shop for groceries, how she enjoyed making salads, how she enjoyed learning how to sew with her mother. She talked about the fact that her mother was always home when she came home from school, that she could trust her mother, that she could depend on her mother, that her mother was there when she needed her. She shared with me some experiences she had had discussing situations that occurred in school, where kids had been teasing her, and how she was able to talk about those experiences with her mother.

Ms. Tucker: Now, as to Calvin—they call him Cal, don't they?

Dr. Benedek: Yes.

Ms. Tucker: Cal is six, right?

Dr. Benedek: Yes.

Ms. Tucker: And what kind of examination did you undertake with Cal?

Dr. Benedek: Cal is a very young child, and so I did a somewhat different evaluation with Cal. The older children were able to talk about their feelings. Cal was able in some ways to talk but also to play out some of his concerns. So, I did an evaluation which contained some talking and some questioning and some playing with Cal.

Ms. Tucker: And what were the results of this examination?

Dr. Benedek: As I indicated earlier, Mrs. Smith told me that Cal had had some difficulties in school. He had some problems paying attention, sitting still; he had problems with his handwriting, his fine motor coordination; he had a lot of trouble paying attention. There had been a diagnosis made in the past and Cal was under psychiatric care. My evaluation of Cal substantiated those impressions. After seeing him, I felt relatively certain that he ought to continue in psychiatric care. Cal told me about the fact that he had spent a lot of time with his father recently, and, in fact, he showed me some of the things that his father had given him, such as a belt buckle with a Lone Star on it made out of gold. He discussed a 10-speed bike that his father had given him.

Ms. Tucker: Excuse me, Doctor. Have the gifts increased, according to the children, since the litigation got under way?

Dr. Benedek: Yes, counsel. All of the children indicated that there have been a great many gifts. . . .

Mr. Specia: Objection, Your Honor, I think this is irrelevant.

Judge Haberman: Overruled.

Ms. Tucker: Thank you, Your Honor. Doctor, I will repeat the question. Does it appear from what you have heard from the family that the gifts emanating from Mr. Smith have increased?

Dr. Benedek: Yes. All of the children told me that their father had been much more generous and, in fact, the older boy was quite concerned about how his father could afford all these nifty presents. In addition, all of the children told me about a trip to Disneyland—the first vacation that they have had with their father—and a promised trip to Bermuda.

Ms. Tucker: Wow! *(laughter in courtroom)* So let me wind up very quickly. The last person in the family that you saw was Lula Bell Jones, is that correct?

Dr. Benedek: Yes, counsel, that is correct.

Ms. Tucker: And she is the maternal grandmother?

Dr. Benedek: Yes, counsel.

Ms. Tucker: All right. Did she give you any insight as to the problems in the Smith home?

Dr. Benedek: Yes, she did. She was quite open and honest about the fact that her daughter, under stress, resorted to alcohol to self-medicate herself. She indicated, though, that she had not seen her daughter drinking in the past several years and, in fact, had not seen any liquor in the house; that she had an opportunity to be in the house quite a bit, since she assumes responsibility for caring for the children when the mother thinks she's going to be late or unavailable.

Ms. Tucker: In your opinion, is Mrs. Jones an adequate mother substitute, an aide to the mother in care for the children?

Dr. Benedek: Yes, in my opinion, Lula Bell Jones is a great deal of help and support to the mother, and she is willing to provide care for the children when the mother is not available.

Ms. Tucker: Thank you, Doctor. I'll pass the witness for now.

Mr. Specia: Doctor Benedek, that was a rather glowing report relating to Joan Smith. Are you at all concerned about her drinking problem?

Dr. Benedek: Yes, counsel, I am concerned. However, at this point in time, it seems to me that Mrs. Smith has taken appropriate measures to seek help for her drinking problem.

Mr. Specia: How long has she been in therapy for alcoholism?

Dr. Benedek: She has been going to Alcoholics Anonymous for the past three months, and on two occasions in the past, after her hospitalizations, she attended Alcoholics Anonymous.

Dr. Specia: Are you aware of the high rate of recidivism in alcoholic treatment?

Dr. Benedek: Yes, counsel, I am.

Mr. Specia: When Joan Smith is drinking heavily, can she provide a home for these children?

Dr. Benedek: There were two occasions, as I mentioned, when Mrs. Smith was drinking heavily. The younger children were not aware of her drinking. The older boy was aware of her drinking on one occasion. He indicated, though, that despite the fact that his mother was drinking, she was always in the home; she cooked all the meals; she was available to talk to him if he had things to talk about. She was never absent from him psychologically, and he described what he meant. He indicated that that was very different from his father who, despite the fact. . . .

Mr. Specia: Excuse me, let me ask you a question. Was the mother in the room when you asked these questions?

Dr. Benedek: With the boy?

Mr. Specia: Yes.

Dr. Benedek: Yes; I'm trying to remember if, in fact, she was in the room. I did interview the mother and all the children together, and I think we did talk about the mother's drinking problems when the mother was in the room. Yes, counsel.

Mr. Specia: It would be very difficult for the young man, then, not to defend his mother, wouldn't it?

Dr. Benedek: We talked about it when she was not in the room also. We talked about it on two occasions.

Mr. Specia: Are you concerned about her promiscuity in front of the children?

Dr. Benedek: Sir, I do not know anything about that.

Mr. Specia: There is evidence in the record that she has been carrying on with other men in front of the children. How does that affect your diagnosis?

Dr. Benedek: All right; I discussed Mrs. Smith's dating patterns with her at length and with the children, and she indicated she had been dating other men, that she had talked with the children about the fact that she would be going out, and the children shared the fact that they were concerned about that and worried. She denied any sexual activity in front of the children, and the children did not give any evidence of men staying in the house overnight.

Mr. Specia: Mrs. Smith is not yet divorced. Do you see any problem with her dating prior to the divorce and confusing the children?

Dr. Benedek: No, counsel, I do not. Especially since Mrs. Smith has spent a great deal of time talking with the children about the fact that she is going out with other men, and that these men are friends of hers.

Mr. Specia: You described her as being mildly depressed at this point. Is depression the type of mental illness that goes in cycles?

Dr. Benedek: In this particular case, I think Mrs. Smith's depression is reactive to the divorce, the new responsibilities and new roles she will have to assume. Depression in other instances may be a cyclic phenomenon, but in this particular case, I don't think it is.

Mr. Specia: Well, how did the two prior hospitalizations for depression fit into your diagnosis?

Dr. Benedek: Mrs. Smith told me that there were serious problems, marital problems, around the time the children were conceived; that the pregnancies were unwanted and unplanned, and that she had expected to be able to go to college. In addition, her husband had begun to physically abuse her. She said that on each of these occasions she felt trapped and very unhappy, and the depressions were reactive to her situation.

Mr. Specia: You are very optimistic, then, about her not only being able to deal with her depression but with her drinking problem at the same time?

Dr. Benedek: Yes, counsel, I am optimistic.

Mr. Specia: What about the additional stresses of being a single parent? How are these going to impact on her depression and her drinking?

Dr. Benedek: I think Mrs. Smith has spent a great deal of time talking with people and thinking about how she will adjust to a new role of a single parent. She has a great deal of support in her family. Her mother and her father spend time with her and with the children. She has a network of support. She belongs to a single-parent group, where the single parents discuss these issues at great length. She's sought out these contacts in the community by herself, recognizing that she will have problems in this new role, and I think that's indicative of a great deal of strength on her part.

Mr. Specia: Doctor, you seem to criticize Mr. Smith for crying in front of his children. It seems like, on one hand, we're calling him an obsessive-compulsive personality, but when he starts responding to feelings, he's being criticized for it.

Dr. Benedek: Sir, I was simply describing Mr. Smith's behavior.

Mr. Specia: What are the nature of Calvin's psychiatric problems?

Dr. Benedek: Calvin was described by his mother as a youngster who had a great deal of difficulty sitting still, paying attention, concentrating. Behaviorally, she describes Calvin as simply not even being able to pay attention to a program on television. He's having a great deal of trouble in the first grade in school. He can hardly write his name. This information was corroborated by my evaluation of Calvin and in material that I had obtained from the physician who was treating Calvin.

Mr. Specia: Might Mrs. Smith's not being a consistent parent add to this problem?

Dr. Benedek: Certainly that's correct, although I would not characterize her as a nonconsistent parent.

Mr. Specia: Well, we have evidence both ways on that. Is there something wrong with the father trying to give to his children and do nice things for them?

Dr. Benedek: There is nothing wrong with the father, a father, giving to children. However, the nature of Mr. Smith's gifts indicate to me that he is more comfortable giving in one way than another. That is to say, he's very comfortable being extremely generous, giving material gifts, but he's not so comfortable giving in a way that is more important to children, that is, giving love, affection and care.

Mr. Specia: Excuse me. Do you have anything positive to say about Mr. Smith? (*laughter in courtroom*)

Dr. Benedek: Counsel, would you tell me what you mean particularly? Or ask me a question?

Mr. Specia: Well, I would just like to know—it seems that you've charted Mrs. Smith as a consistent, loving, warm parent and given Mr. Smith very little credit for his role in the family. Do you see any of his qualities as being beneficial in a parent?

Dr. Benedek: Yes; I think Mr. Smith has a great many good characteristics. He indicates that he's interested in his children, that he wants to spend time with them, and that he wants to change his patterns of behavior. I am very concerned, however, about the fact that Mr. Smith, although saying that he thinks it's important that Calvin have psychiatric care, is currently not willing to pay for such care for Calvin.

Mr. Specia: Doctor, are you a mother?

Dr. Benedek: Yes, sir, I am.

Mr. Specia: Do you think that your being a mother might affect your professional opinion in a case like this?

Dr. Benedek: I think that being a mother may affect my professional opinion. However, in this particular case I think it's very clear that the mother would be acting in the best interest of the children, and I do not think the fact that I am a mother has influenced my opinions in this particular case.

Mr. Specia: I pass the witness, Your Honor.

Judge Haberman: Ms. Tucker?

Ms. Tucker: Doctor, how would you compare the validity of the testimony of an expert witness, such as yourself, who has seen the whole family and the validity of an expert who has seen only one member of the family?

Mr. Specia: Objection, Your Honor. *(laughter in courtroom)* Determining the validity and the ways of an expert's testimony is within the purview of the Court, and I don't think she should be permitted to testify to this.

Judge Haberman: Sustained, counsel.

Ms. Tucker: Thank you, Your Honor. But you have seen the way that the Smith family group interacted?

Dr. Benedek: Yes, counsel. I have had the opportunity to interview Mr. Smith, Mrs. Smith, all the Smith children and Mrs. Smith's mother and to watch the mother and the father interact with the children in my office.

Ms. Tucker: The mother, the three children and the grandmother. What was your opinion as to the quality of this group's functioning at the present time.

Dr. Benedek: It was my opinion, based on my observations, that the quality of functioning of the mother, the grandmother, and the children were unimpaired, with the exception of the fact that Calvin does have a psychiatric difficulty.

Ms. Tucker: Now we've heard much talk at this point about Joan's past history of drinking. Doctor, isn't it true that most families today are dealing with some sort of stress?

Dr. Benedek: Yes, counsel, that is correct. Many families are dealing with stress.

Ms. Tucker: At this point, is it true that Joan is coping well with the stress that she finds herself under?

Dr. Benedek: Yes; it's my impression that Mrs. Smith is coping very actively with the stress that she finds herself under and in a very appropriate manner.

Ms. Tucker: Is it your opinion that the children are having their needs met at the present time in the Smith home?

Dr. Benedek: Yes, counsel; it's my opinion that the children who are currently living with Mrs. Smith are having their needs met, and the children very clearly expressed to me the fact that they were happy, content, and wanted to live with their mother.

Ms. Tucker: Given the two parents with whom you are familiar, who, in your expert opinion, do you feel is better able to provide a loving, stable home for the three children?

Dr. Benedek: It is my opinion that, at this point in time, the mother, Mrs. Smith, is able to provide for the children in the best way.

Ms. Tucker: And you are certain of this?

Dr. Benedek: Yes, counsel, I am.

Ms. Tucker: Thank you. Pass.

Judge Haberman: That's it?

Ms. Tucker: Yes, we're over, as it is.

Judge Haberman: You are resting your case?

Ms. Tucker: Yes, we close.

Judge Haberman: We thank you for your testimony, and you may join the others either out in the hall, or, if you would like to listen to arguments which follow in this case, you may come back into the courtroom and be with us during the argument stage.

[*to the audience*] Ladies and gentlemen, generally we have perhaps even additional witnesses or rebuttal witnesses in many cases. After this, we hear arguments from counsel. And, in many instances, the court may determine whether it be best to visit with one of the children or, for that matter, all three of the children. In this particular case, I would assume that some of the other witnesses would have caused other concerns for the Court to consider. Many times, the attorneys will request that the Court have an interview with one, two, or the three children involved. In this particular case, I probably would have had an additional interview with the oldest child, at least. However, it probably would have been dependent on what the other witnesses would have brought out in testimony.

It is pretty clear to me that, at this point, hearing what we have just heard here, I would keep all three children together, and that, in Texas, the mother would become the managing conservator. However, much of this would have been dependent upon an interview with the oldest child. If that interview with the oldest child had shed additional light on some of the reasons why the boy wanted to live with his father at this time, I would have seriously considered the oldest child going with the father—not at this particular moment, because of his tax season and other responsibilities, but perhaps starting at the end of school. Judges often think about things in terms of school periods, because we don't want to transfer children from one school to another school if not really necessary. Therefore, in talking with the child, I would have considered his school system. But just from what we have heard from the two witnesses, I don't have any additional information to offer on that. I would probably, in this case, leave the three children together with the mother at this time. I would perhaps have given the father somewhat more expanded visitation rights than in our usual standard case.

I really think that the father may well be an exceptionally fine resource for these children, but I would have liked to hear additional testimony as to the duration of some of his commitments. In other words, if the Kiwanis Club and the other commitments are just for this year, it would perhaps have made a difference in my estimation, mainly regarding the oldest child, as to whether or not the father would have that child, starting in the September school period, after a visitation period during the summer.

These, then, are the types of considerations that we see in most situations now. I want to tell you, these were very calm, cool, and collected attorneys, compared to those in the average custody situation. We do have joint custody in Texas, and sometimes the parties can agree to joint custody. In other words, the court can approve joint custody plans for children in Texas. However, if the parties could not agree to this, then the court must choose one over the other as managing conservator.

Part IV

ETHICAL ISSUES

9

The Responsibilities of Psychiatrists to Society

Paul Chodoff, M.D.

American psychiatrists as individuals are responsible to the society which they serve and which sanctions their activities. The nature of this responsibility can be subsumed under the following headings:

1) *The responsibility of citizenship.* The psychiatrist in the role of citizen has multiple responsibilities. He/she is required to act in a useful and informed manner in the general society, to share special knowledge with the public, and to make his/her voice heard in the public discussion and determination of issues which are of legitimate interest to psychiatry. The psychiatrist also has the responsibility to establish, maintain, and adhere to standards of professional integrity.

2) *The responsibility to be accountable to the public and its representatives.*

3) *The responsibility to assist in promoting an equitable distribution of psychiatric services throughout the entire socio-economic range of American society.*

It is self-evident that psychiatrists should behave in a decent, law-abiding fashion. Like other well-educated citizens occupying a favored position in society, the psychiatrist ought to devote some time and effort to an informed participation in the affairs of community and nation. We should remember, however, that our crystal ball is likely to be as clouded as anyone else's and that our special training does not make us instant experts on everything that goes on in the world. Psychiatrists may be particularly susceptible to this hubristic temptation because of the intense relationships which they develop with patients and because of the illusion of omnipotence, an occupational hazard (1). On the other hand, some practitioners believe that any activity which exposes them to public scrutiny compromises their relationship with their patients. Such a belief, when genuinely held, merits respect.

Do psychiatrists have the responsibility to respond to questions asked by legitimate organs of public information about subjects thought to relate to their field? Such questions often run the gamut, reflecting a popular belief in the seer-like qualities of our profession, a belief that represents only one side of an ambivalence which also sees us as bombastic simpletons. We may be asked to comment on issues ranging from the political misuse of psychiatry to the psychology of gasoline lines. When queried in this fashion, the individual psychiatrist should, in my view, respond substantively only if he feels that he has an opinion worth expressing about the subject. He should make it clear that his opinion is his own and that he does not speak for a professional organization, unless of course he is acting as an official spokesman. In any event, he should eschew broad and specious generalizations. I refer here to such disasters as the 1964 poll in which a number of psychiatrists expressed an adverse opinion about Barry Goldwater's mental health. Another such instance, and one which unfortunately is rather popular at present, concerns certain "psychobiographies" undertaken by psychiatrists or written with their aid, which dissect public figures in painful and embarrassing ways on the basis of little or no direct data. Although one cannot deny that it is the privilege of some psychiatrists to make fools of themselves, to do so certainly does not constitute a responsibility to society. Indeed, the responsibility here is to avoid such self-serving and publicity-seeking fiascos.

Does a psychiatrist have the responsibility to voice his/her opinion when it is contrary to that officially put forward by the professional organizations which represent him/her? I believe that in such instances, the psychiatrist has a responsibility to consider the opposition seriously and to take into account the possible effects of stating a divergent opinion. Extreme and intransigent statements may do a good deal of harm to the reputation and interests of the profession, and also may produce confusion in the public. On the other hand, the individual psychiatrist certainly is not compelled to align him/herself slavishly with positions to which he/she has strong objections. Differing opinions need to be voiced, and, if well reasoned, they should be treated respectfully by other psychiatrists and by psychiatric organizations. Even if they do not result in a change or modification of the opposed position they should be received without a responsive invective that demeans the profession and confuses the public.

Psychiatrists certainly have a responsibility to take part in the activities of the professional organizations which represent them to the public, and they should lend their voices in a democratic fashion to the formulation of professional policy. This is the first level at which differing points of view need to be aired and resolved to the degree possible. As is true of all organizations composed of members who participate in their activities in widely varying degrees, accusations of cliquishness and hierarchical domination come with little grace from those who satisfy only the formal and minimal requirements of membership.

In the case of issues which have to be dealt with at an organizational rather than an individual level, we are faced with a different level of responsibility—that of the profession itself. These responsibilities will be dealt with by Dr. Michels in Chapter 10.

My remarks about the responsibility of the psychiatrist as citizen have thus far, I believe, been relatively unexceptionable. The need to understand the relationship between responsibilities to society and to the profession, may however, involve the psychiatrist in more ambiguous decisions. It is a hallmark of psychiatry that in a number of areas (e.g., involuntary hospitalization, the insanity defense) the psychiatrist operates at an interface between the rights of the individual and the requirements of society. Thus, a psychiatrist is particularly vulnerable to state and cultural influences. Instances will arise when such influences come into conflict with professional convictions. On such occasions, the sometimes difficult issue to be faced is whether true responsibility to society necessitates adherence to professional standards or to societal dictates.

Especially with regard to improper state or governmental attempts to influence decisions, the threat to the psychiatrist's professional integrity is likely to be more serious in totalitarian than in democratic countries. We have seen a particularly heinous example in the Soviet Union of how psychiatry can be perverted under state pressure to suppress political dissent. For a number of reasons inherent in the structure of our society, it is improbable that we will be faced with such extreme efforts to compromise our professional integrity. This does not mean, however, that problems similar in type but subtler in nature cannot occur in our country, particularly among psychiatrists employed at various governmental levels. Examples include state hospital psychiatrists acceding without protest to inadequate standards of care, or holding on to patients for too long, or, more likely today, too short a period of time in response to outside pressure. Considerations other than the patients' real needs may influence the treatment decisions of psychiatrists in the military or in prison systems.

Private practitioners of psychiatry are less susceptible to governmental pressure. However, all psychiatrists, not only in this country but everywhere, and not only those receiving salaries in organized settings, operate within the confines of a cultural net which exerts a pervasive though sometimes unnoticed effect on their judgments. For example, psychiatrists have written letters (before the easing of restrictions) to legitimize claims for abortion on the grounds of a nonexistent or very tenuous suicidal tendency, or to secure draft deferments during the Vietnam war because of nonexistent mental illness. I submit that in such cases, as well as in the case of state pressure on institutional psychiatrists, all of us must seriously face the question of whether we are compromising our real responsibility to society when we bend or ignore the ethical standards of our profession even in a cause which we consider a good one.

I turn now to a discussion of responsibility as accountability. In recent years, there has been an upsurge of interest in accountability stemming mainly from two factors. First, there is the effect of the burgeoning consumer movement—Naderism—which requires that the purveyor of any goods or services must be accountable to the public. This means that he/she must provide answers to questions about the scope, legitimacy, and effectiveness of the operations for which he/she receives payment and he/she must provide machinery for redress of errors or wrongs. Second is the impact of the introduction of payment by a third party (usually commercial and doctor-sponsored health insurance companies) on the services rendered by psychiatrists, particularly those working in the private sector (2). These two complementary influences have induced considerable unrest among psychiatrists and an increasing amount of responsive activity. They have also been responsible for a serious conflict between the values inherent in the concept of accountability and the values of confidentiality as manifested in the patient-psychiatrist relationship. I shall have more to say about this conflict.

The concept of accountability, however, has much earlier historical roots and a more general application than the above. In explanation, I go back to a time when philosophers debated how kings and lords could be controlled and held responsible (3). By contracting to be ruled, did the people thereby abrogate their right to any accounting for the power which they had turned over to the ruler? This is what Hobbes thought, and it is a doctrine also manifested as the divine right of kings: the king being accountable only to God, while the sole resource of the people was to petition and pray. The doctrine opposing this absolutist view holds that the monarch is a representative of the people, that he receives his power from the people and is accountable to them. In modern societies, of course, the latter theory has achieved primacy to such an extent that even in totalitarian regimes it is paid lip-service by dictators. The world now being in a relatively short supply of monarchs, the present application of this ancient debate is that those who wield significant power must account for it. Thus, in this country and in other democracies, the holders of governmental power must explain themselves endlessly and justify their actions to their constituents. This is true, however, not only for politicians; it also holds to varying degrees for educators, corporate officers, researchers, football coaches, etc.; and I believe that this equation of power-responsibility-accountability also applies to psychiatrists. Jonas Robitscher (4) has gone so far as to assert that the psychiatrist has become the most important non-governmental decision-maker in modern life, disposing, in fact, of more power than most governmental officials. Robitscher views this state of affairs with alarm. He feels that psychiatric power is not subject to public scrutiny, enlightening review, constitutional limitations or even, sometimes, personal protest. In short, he sees the psychiatrists as operating in relative immunity from the necessity to account for themselves. Without fully endorsing Robitscher's view, I believe that we must acknowledge that psychiatrists exert a significant influence in many areas of public life as well as in the lives of their patients, and that possibly they have been insufficiently responsive to the public in accounting for this influence. I propose also to explore the responsibility of psychiatrists to be accountable in this broader use of the term.

To return to the confidentiality-accountability conflict, all of us would agree that one of the values which makes the profession of psychiatry unique is the ability of its practitioners to promise their patients that information transmitted in the course of the therapeutic encounter will be inviolate. In recent years, there has been an increasing uneasiness about the sanctity of this contract. The threat comes from two sources. First has been the advent of new methods of payment for psychiatric services necessitating the transmission of diagnostic information about patients to insurance companies (2). The fact that this development has occurred at a time when individuals in our society feel almost overwhelmed by bureaucratic and technological dominance has augmented the uneasiness. No one can be certain that patient information will be safe from disclosure when disseminated within vast and impersonal networks. The second threat to psychiatric confidentiality has emerged in the legal arena, as the psychiatrist has also become concerned about the privacy of records about patients. A host of legal decisions has penetrated the psychiatrist-patient privilege, whether this is in the control of the patient alone, as is usually the case, or also of the psychiatrist, as in Illinois and Wisconsin. It is questionable whether the recently enacted psychotherapist-patient privilege will protect confidentiality effectively (5). Thus, psychiatrists are confronted with a serious challenge to their ability to resist demands that they reveal intimate knowledge about their patients in court.

Certainly psychiatrists have reason to be concerned about these threats to confidentiality.* They have reacted vigorously and appropriately through formation of the National Commission on Confidentiality of Health Records and espousal of psychotherapist-patient privilege laws. I am, however, concerned that in our eagerness to rally to the banner of confidentiality, we may be doing less than full justice to our responsibility to be accountable for the services we render to those who are paying for them. We need to keep in mind the great difference between a two-party contract, in which the therapist need account only to the patient for what transpires between the two (with the exception, of course, of illegal and fraudulent practices), and a three-party contract, where payment funds come from pools of subscriber money and to some extent and probably increasingly in the future, from governmental contributions (2). Such third-party carriers have not only the right but the duty to be provided enough information to protect themselves and their subscribers from overutilization, fraud, abuse, and misuse of the services their subscribers are paying for. Without a reasonable amount of relevant information, they are handicapped in their rational efforts to plan and project

---

* Other opinions have been expressed. Modlin (6) suggests that patient-psychiatrist confidentiality is of more concern to the former than the latter.

their operations and to insulate their subscribers from crippling expenses. Since these benefits make needed psychiatric services available to a wider socioeconomic range, it is in the public interest as well as in the interests of psychiatrists to cooperate in making these third-party operations successful.

While a minority of psychiatrists challenge the need to transmit any diagnostic information at all to insurance companies, most will acknowledge their responsibility to do so. However, it appears that their apparent acceptance is often more formal or verbal than genuine, and in fact the resistance to conveying patient information is deep-seated. Such resistance is always justified on the grounds that disclosure poses a threat to the patient's interests or to the therapeutic relationship.

Certainly we must be alert to minimize the real possibility that intrusive insurance interferences may cause damage. However, I question whether the available evidence indicates that such instances have been so numerous or devastating as to warrant serious alarm at the possibility of a complete destruction of confidentiality through insurance requirements. For example, in the case of the extensive psychiatric coverage provided by Blue Shield and Blue Cross in Washington, D.C., under the Federal Employee Benefit Program, there have been no authenticated cases in which psychiatric information has been improperly disseminated (7). The dangers to confidentiality from fiscal third parties are real, but they can be overemphasized—even to the point of becoming a shibboleth.

I feel that both our professional interests and our responsibility to society require us to examine the possibility that the third-party threat to confidentiality is being exaggerated. I shall support this contention by listing a number of reasons other than confidentiality considerations which may be making us reluctant to transmit information to insurance companies. First, as citizens living in an increasingly interdependent and technological society, we share the general revulsion at the specter of Big Brother brooding over and monitoring our every activity, even the most private ones. Then, we are also physicians, and physicians, particularly private practitioners, tend to be a tetchy and individualistic lot, intent on protecting their essentially entrepreneurial activities from supervision or interference by anyone else, even from those paying the bills. Also, psychiatrists are a rather special variety of physician. Our relationship with third-party carriers is different from those of other physicians. We believe, and with some justification, that we are regarded with suspicion by the insurance companies and are being asked to divulge more information about our patients and treatment plans than that required from other specialties. Finally, those of us who practice in primarily psychoanalytic and psychotherapeutic modes must deal with the reality that a certain number of our patients, while presenting significant psychopathology or serious problem in living, simply do not fit medical diagnostic criteria very well. Therefore we may feel some uneasiness and even defensiveness about the whole process of diagnosis. We may fear that our problems in conforming to this aspect of the medical model will jeopardize the coverage of our patients or limit the amount of treatment authorized.

In short, I am suggesting that our preoccupation with confidentiality in regard to insurance transactions is overdone—and that it contains elements of rationalization fueled by the above motivations.

We live in a changing society, which is successfully demanding alterations in the way medical care, including that provided by psychiatrists, is being paid for. Certainly, we need to protect the interests of our patients and our efforts to help them. But both our patients and ourselves have to face the fact that the requirement that we be accountable to third parties is increasing in scope and is inherently incompatible with absolute confidentiality. To fight too hard, on the basis of somewhat suspect motives, for an unattainable purity of confidentiality may be self-defeating. In the long run, it will not serve the interests of our patients or of a society moving towards an egalitarian ideal.

Thus far, I have been discussing the conflict between confidentiality and accountability as it is affected by third-party payment for psychiatric services. I have previously indicated that therapist-patient confidentiality is also threatened by demands for information about patients from courts and law enforcement agencies. Here we enter a difficult and painful area and one which is presently enmeshed in a thicket of unresolved judicial decisions. I can understand the tenacity with which certain psychiatrists have resisted such demands for information. I admire their willingness even to go to prison to support their principles. Certainly, it is the responsibility of the psychiatrist, like any other citizen, to obey the laws and judicial decrees. However, as I have previously indicated, a psychiatrist may find himself in circumstances where he believes that he can discharge his proper responsibility to society only by resisting its dictates if he believes that these are intolerable because they are in conflict with the ethics and values of his profession. Exemplary actions of this kind can have a dramatic effect. However, apart from such exceptional and extreme cases, the tasks of formulating policy and taking action to inform the public and influence legislatures and courts are more appropriately undertaken by psychiatric professional organizations than by individual psychiatrists.

I turn now from consideration of the confidentiality-accountability dilemma to a consideration of accountability in the more general sense alluded to previously: the need for our profession to be accountable for the power which it has been vouchsafed by society. This power is manifested in many ways: in our authority to make certain important decisions involving the lives of our patients and their families; in involuntary commitment procedures; in judicial decisions imputing responsibility for criminal behavior; in methods of treatment, sometimes administered against the will of the recipients and which are potent and have far-reaching and sometimes troubling effects; in research activities involving feeling and behavior; in ventures involving national and international politics; and in the application of diagnostic labels which may profoundly affect the lives of the people to whom they have been affixed.

Certainly, one essential responsibility to the society we serve and which has granted us these powers is the assurance that we are in control of our activities and are effectively policing our ranks. In fact, a profession has been defined as an occupation whose activities are important and which has earned sufficient confidence from the public so that it is allowed to regulate itself (8). Thus, we need to discharge this responsibility by instituting mechanisms to protect the public from a variety of unacceptable practices ranging from the illegal to the improper. Such potential misprisions cover a wide range in accordance with the diverse nature of our activities. Examples include obviously heinous behavior such as the sexual seduction of a patient under the masquerade of therapy; acts of deception and collusion for financial gain (incidentally, there is more opportunity for these to occur in connection with three-party than two-party payment systems (9)); abuse, misuse, or overutilization of legitimate treatment modalities; practicing with improper or insufficient qualifications or under the handicap of incapacitating physical or mental illness. In such instances, the responsibility of the individual psychiatrist does not lie in taking personal corrective or disciplinary action. Clearly this is beyond his province and falls within the scope of professional organizations through their Ethics or Peer Review Committees (10), or law enforcement agencies. It is, however, the responsibility of individual psychiatrists to bring the questionable behavior of their colleagues to the attention of those empowered to deal with them. This is usually a hard duty and can be an agonizing one. Uncertainty about the facts as well as motives, both friendly and humanitarian, towards the involved practitioner may stand in our way. What do we do, for instance, when we learn that an admired and esteemed colleague has developed such a failing of powers as a result of the aging process that he/she is no longer competent to treat patients? Here too, as well as in other instances of illegal, unethical, or incompetent behavior on the part of our fellow psychiatrists, we may find ourselves in a conflict between the value of confidentiality and the duty to protect both the public and the good name of our profession (11). Obviously, when confronted with such a decision, we must be guided by ethical principles and by a consideration of all the factors involved in a complicated situation. As experts, however, in the multifarious ways in which human beings disguise their behavior and deceive themselves

236 Law and Ethics in the Practice of Psychiatry

about their motives, we need to keep alert to the possibility that we may avoid taking a responsible action because it is difficult or painful.

While there may well be differences about means, no reputable psychiatrist will take issue with the principle that the profession must regulate itself and that individual practitioners should participate appropriately in the regulating process. However, I do not believe that our responsibility to society in response to the power vested in us ends with the detection and correction of instances of neglect, abuse, or malfeasance.

I believe that proper accountability also means that we have an obligation to present to the public a reasonably coherent picture of the nature, scope, effectiveness and limitations of the profession of psychiatry. How do we resemble and differ from allied mental health professions? From other medical practitioners? What sorts of conditions do we deal with among our patients? Ought we to undertake the care and cure of society as well as of individuals? How effective are our psychotherapeutic efforts? These questions and others like them cause legitimate confusion among the informed laity who are concerned with our activities. The reasons for this state of affairs is to some extent inherent in the nature of our profession, a reflection of the fact that we are required to maintain as best we can an uneasy balance, with one foot in biological medicine and the other in social concerns. There are, however, other, more immediate reasons for the identity crisis of psychiatry which we hear so much about nowadays. The inherent problem has been compounded by real differences within our ranks, by conflicts of direction and interest, and these differences are being accentuated by the impact of the rapidly changing times in which we live. A factor of particular importance is the potential impact of the new third-party methods of payment for our services (2). It is disturbingly possible that these differences may harden into a schism in our ranks between the "doctors" and the "psychotherapists."

This crisis of professional identity cannot be regarded entirely in a negative way. To some extent it constitutes a sign of health and vigor in response to the social changes which affect us. But it needs to be dealt with, not only to protect the future of our profession, but also to enable us better to help the public understand the nature of the services we render, our qualifications for exercising the power that we possess and the knowledge that we have accumulated.

Our responsibility to society in this respect will not be discharged by official proclamations or committee reports. At the present stage, when we are lacking a consensus about how to answer the many vexing questions facing us, pronouncements from on high can be only a papering-over or an exercise in premature closure. I believe that we can best deal with the uncertain state in which our profession now finds itself by frank and candid discussions among psychiatrists and by efforts on the part of individuals to think through the issues involved and to present the fruit of their reflections to their colleagues. An admirable example of such a discussion dealing with the role of psychiatrists in the ills of society was given by Gerald Klerman in an NIMH Staff College lecture last Spring (12). Such a course, that of an open exchange of opinions, is in the best democratic tradition. As psychiatry responds to changing conditions, it is up to us not only to guide these changes as wisely as possible, but also to let the public know what is happening so that it can know what to expect from us.

In this presentation, I have dealt with the first two areas of responsibility of psychiatrists and psychiatry to our society; namely, the responsibility of citizenship and the responsibility to be accountable to the public. The third responsibility—to foster distributive justice about the allocation of the resources at our disposal—can be discharged effectively only by actions taken by the profession as a whole rather than by individual psychiatrists. I should like to emphasize, however, that all psychiatrists need to maintain an awareness of the importance of this responsibility not only because we owe it to our society but also because it constitutes one aspect of the concern for the welfare of other people which played a role in our decision to devote our professional lives to psychiatry.

REFERENCES

1. Marmor, J.: The feeling of superiority: An occupational hazard in the practice of psychotherapy. *Am. J. Psychiat.,* 110:370-376, 1953-4.
2. Chodoff, P.: Psychiatry and the fiscal third party. *Am. J. Psychiat.,* 135: 10, pp. 497-510, Oct., 1978.
3. Sibley, M. Q.: *Political Ideas and Ideologies.* New York-Evanston-London: Harper & Row, 1970.
4. Robitscher, J.: *The Powers of Psychiatry.* Boston: Houghton-Mifflin Co., 1980.
5. Slovenko, R.: Accountability and abuse of psychiatric confidentiality. Presented at Third Annual International Symposium on Law and Psychiatry, British Columbia, Canada, May 10-13, 1979.
6. Modlin, H. C.: How private is privacy? *Psychiatry Digest,* Vol. 30, 13-17, Feb., 1969.
7. Adland, M.: Personal communication. Psychiatric Consultant to Group Hospitalization of D.C.
8. Freidson, E.: *Profession of Medicine.* New York: Dodd, Mead and Co., 1972.
9. Towery, O. B. and Sharfstein, S. S.: Fraud and abuse in psychiatric practice. *Am. J. Psychiat.,* 135:1, pp. 92-94, Jan., 1978.
10. Chodoff, P.: Psychiatric peer review: The Washington, D.C. experience, 1972-1975. *Am. J. Psychiat.,* 134:2, pp. 121-125, Feb., 1977.
11. Doyle, B. B.: Psychiatric illness in physicians: Confidentiality vs. responsibility. Presented at a special session on "The Impaired Physician," Annual Meeting of the American Psychiatric Association, Atlanta, Ga., May 10, 1978.
12. Klerman, G. L.: The limits of mental health. Presented as Staff College Lecture, NIMH, June 13, 1979.

10

The Responsibility of Psychiatry to Society

Robert Michels, M.D.

Dr. Chodoff indicated that one of the responsibilities of individual psychiatrists is "to take part in the activities of the professional organizations which represent them to the public and . . . lend their voices in a democratic fashion to the formulation of professional policy" (1). This statement recognizes that psychiatrists, like other physicians, are more than healers; they are professional healers. They recognize the importance of a peer constituency as well as a client constitutency. As an organized profession, psychiatrists have a collective responsibility to society in addition to their individual responsibility as practitioners. Before discussing the responsibilities of psychiatry as a profession, I should like to offer some introductory comments on professions in general and on ethics by quoting from a previous essay of mine dealing with this subject.

PROFESSIONS AND ETHICS

The *Oxford English Dictionary* defines a profession as "a vocation in which professed knowledge of some department of learning or science is used in its application to the affairs of others or in the practice of an art founded upon it." Traditionally the term has been applied to divinity, law and medicine. Freidson, the medical sociologist, points out the dual meaning of profession as a special kind of occupation and as an avowal or promise. He defines a profession as "an occupation which has assumed a dominant position in a division of labor, so that it gains control over the determination of the substance of its own work" (2). Goode identifies the core characteristics of a profession as "a prolonged specialized training in a body of abstract knowledge, and a collectivity or service orientation" (3).

These two themes, relating to knowledge on the one hand and its application in practice on the other, place professions in an intermediate position between sciences and trades, but differentiate them from both. Trades do not stem from abstract knowledge but from commercial interest, and they make no pretense at an ethic which places the general good or public service above their parochial concerns. Perhaps it would be more accurate to say that when they do make such pretenses, few take them seriously. In recent years, some social critics have urged trades to be more professional, to show more concern with broad social issues. Interestingly, they are often the same critics who have attacked professional organizations for pretending to moral leadership, arguing that their appropriate function is that of a trade union.

Pure science is the pursuit of knowledge without regard to its application. There is a critical difference between professional and scientific activity. Science is radical or revolutionary, forever trying new methods, questioning accepted views and rejecting arguments from established authority. Professions are inherently conservative, preferring the tested and traditional. Thus, our standards for accepting a new drug are more rigorous than those with which we test a familiar one, while our standards for new or old models of atomic structure are identical. We admire an astronomer who announces that he is testing a new theory concerning the atmosphere of Venus, but regard with mistrust a surgeon who is experimenting with a new method for treating schizophrenia. When our lives or our bodies are at risk, the dangers of error are so great that we are likely to be most cautious before taking the risk of being wrong. The dangers associated with a new idea in science may also be great, but there is usually little difficulty separating them from the mere exploration and testing of the idea. This difference extends to the psychological set of the scientist and the professional while they carry out their daily activities. We expect a good scientist to understand why he is using a certain concentration of reagent in his test tube, and are not overly concerned if he makes an occasional error calculating the formula, as long as he understands the theory behind the calculation. We expect a good physician not to make errors in dosage of a drug, they are too dangerous; although we might not be overly concerned if he has forgotten the theoretical basis for calculating the dosage, as long as he remembers the result.

In a sense, a profession can be seen as a group of people to whom society has delegated power and authority based on the assumption that they have certain knowledge and skills which are not generally available and which are required for decisions in a certain area. Since many of these decisions involve values as well as scientific or technologic considerations, the profession becomes, in effect, a group of ethical as well as scientific specialists. Generally these ethical functions are concealed and there is a pretense that the decisions are really technical or scientific. For example, decisions concerning the distribution of scarce life preserving resources, such as artificial kidneys or rare medicines, are usually rationalized in biotechnologic terms. The reason for this is clear: scientific knowledge itself does not confer ethical sensitivity, and this "generalization of expertise" (4) from scientific to moral, when it is exposed, is an important source of anti-professionalism. I believe that this complaint is often reasonable but the problem is more complex than this brief outline would suggest. It is true that scientific knowledge does not confer ethical expertise, but it may make possible the life experiences which can lead to a refinement of ethical sensitivities. For example, the physician has no special claim to skill in deciding who shall live or who shall die because of his knowledge of anatomy or physiology. However, his knowledge of these fields may have led him to an unusual amount of experience in caring for dying people and may have allowed him that special privilege and responsibility of making scientific or technical decisions which lead to life and death results. Experiences such as these can lead to ethical expertise.

Professionalization, therefore, entails a moral as well as a physical division of labor. Further, every profession involves both license and mandate, and practitioners "by virtue of gaining admission to the charmed circle of the profession, individually exercise a license to do things others do not do, (and) collectively they presume to tell society what is good and right for it in a broad and crucial aspect of life" (5). Professionals are expected to exercise their moral authority not only as individuals, but also as a group when they promote those values for which society has assigned them responsibility (6).

In addition to their knowledge and power, professionals have certain responsibilities — such as the physician's obligation to report certain public health dangers, to provide assistance in emergencies — or, in fact, any of the responsibilities discussed in this volume. Finally, a profession is more than a group; it is an organized collective, and its members function as representatives of the profession accepting their peers' right and duty to define what is acceptable professional behavior. This tradition, stemming from the Hippocratic Code, is so powerful in medicine and psychiatry that it usually resolves any conflict between psychiatrists' obligation to their patients and their obligation to society by imposing an even greater obligation to the ethical code of the profession. This assures the public that such conflicts will be resolved in a consistent way, not according to the individual morality of each specific practitioner (7).

THE GROWTH OF INTEREST IN ETHICS

There has been a striking growth of interest in professional, medical, and psychiatric ethics in recent years. The interest itself is highly desirable, but the factors that have led to it are not all positive. Ethics have to do with human actions, and particularly choices. When there is a consensus about what ought to be done, and when the limiting factor is our capacity to do it, there is much more interest in science and technology than in ethics. This was the situation in medicine and psychiatry only a few decades ago. The picture changes when the consensus about goals breaks down, and when there is no agreement about what would be desirable. It changes even more when the limiting factor in achieving our goals is the availability of resources, and we must set priorities among desirable goals. Science cannot tell us which goals to pursue first and which to defer or even relinquish. Unfortunately, ethics cannot answer these questions either, but they do help us to conduct the dialogue about them in an intelligent way. Ethics help us to discuss values intelligently, but we still must draw on some source of values, such as religion or cultural traditions of humanism, to form a foundation for our goals and choices. Many believe that we are now entering an era of limited resources and a dissolution of the moral consensus that marked the middle third of the century. This has been particularly true in the field of health care, and one consequence has been an increased attention to ethics.

PSYCHIATRY'S RESPONSIBILITIES

A profession is based upon knowledge, and one of the responsibilities of a profession is to nurture, expand, examine, test, and when necessary, reject that knowledge.* In medicine, this has increasingly become the province of academic institutions. As a result, once they have completed their formal training, many members of the profession are relatively isolated from those few who are charged with the responsibility for developing new knowledge. This function is then assigned to a small group of investigators who, in turn, may feel separated from the practitioners. In its extreme form, this leads to a profession that consists not of a united group of learned individuals who share certain core values and advocate certain positions in society, but rather of two quite disparate groups: one seeking to expand and advance knowledge, while holding an almost contemptuous attitude toward the adequacy of the scientific basis of contemporary practice; the other struggling to care for those who need their assistance, suspicious and mistrustful of the damage that might be done to their cause by idealistic scientists who are unfamiliar with the practical problems of applying scientific knowledge.

---

* As the reader will perceive, here I am not using *knowledge* as synonymous with *truth*.

This problem has troubled psychiatry at least as much as other areas of medicine, and is accentuated when there is concern about the distribution of limited resources between research and clinical care. Clearly, there is no simple solution, and yet there are strategies that should be encouraged. The optimal resolution of the profession's problems requires that a dialogue be maintained, and one vital function of the profession is to provide the institutional and social structures that maintain that dialogue. Among the most important are those that maintain the community of the members of the profession—the organizations and journals and meetings that bring the various groups together.

A profession consists of people, and a major responsibility of any profession is its concern that the quality and quantity of its members are appropriate for society's needs. There are a number of ways that this is done. The profession surveys both society and its members to assess the nature of the skills and the number of practitioners needed. It reviews the pool of individuals who seek admission, and when necessary tries to recruit additional applicants. In recent years, this has been a major problem for psychiatry, since it draws upon a small finite group of potential applicants, medical school graduates, and they now perceive it as less attractive relative to their other options than was the case only a few years ago. Psychiatry's responsibility in this instance is increased because there is no sign of significant social or governmental concern about the problem.

A profession generally plays a major role in selecting its members. In the case of psychiatry, this selection occurs in collaboration with the rest of medicine, since for all practical purposes anyone accepted into the medical profession who chooses to become a psychiatrist is free to do so. This means that psychiatry has a responsibility to participate with other medical specialties in the selection of future physicians, since everything we know about the selection of specialties suggests that, if psychiatrists are not involved in the medical school admissions process, even fewer medical students will select psychiatric careers.

After assessing the need for psychiatrists, attracting applicants and selecting among them, the next step is to train them. In psychiatry, this function is distributed between the institutions that develop and conduct training programs and the residency review committees that set standards, review, and accredit them. Training programs are usually embedded in institutions that have major commitments to service, and one problem stems from the fact that the structure and content of their curricula reflect compromises between educational and service goals. This is not necessarily undesirable, but difficulties emerge when resources shrink asymmetrically, and the political process protects service activities with their large immediate constituency more effectively than it protects longer range educational goals. The result may be a distortion of the training program so that it prepares students for practice patterns that reflect the services that are well reimbursed today rather than those the profession believes most relevant for tomorrow. The profession has a responsibility to address this problem, both by advocating public support for its educational goals, and by setting standards for membership that reflect its core values rather than the lowest common denominator of existing training programs. Psychiatry's performance in this regard could be improved; it has not always rejected training programs that were clearly inadequate.

Another responsibility of the profession is to insure that training programs train professionals, not merely practitioners, and that they train them in the responsibilities of their profession. This means that psychiatrists in training must learn more than how to treat patients; they must develop a professional identity and learn the history and the ethical traditions of psychiatry. These are conservative goals, in the literal sense of the word, aimed at conserving social structures that have evolved over many years in order to protect important values. A healer, like a scientist, may be radical or revolutionary, but to some extent a professional must always be conservative. This is not a defense of conservatism, but merely a statement of its logical relationship to professionalism. If a psychiatrist believes that revolutionary goals or methods are desirable or even morally necessary, he should, of course, pursue them. However, he has a responsibility to distinguish these beliefs from his professional values, and to make clear when he speaks as a psychiatrist and when as a citizen who may, at other times, practice psychiatry (8). We have provided little guidance for our trainees in this area. Some of the most gifted and articulate of our colleagues have spoken out on a wide range of social issues, often with both reason and passion, but have done so in a form that suggests that their views should have special consideration because they formerly have been or occasionally are also physicians who treat the mentally ill. The profession has a responsibility, not only to its trainees, but also to the public, to make clear that, whether we individually agree or disagree with their views, we collectively recognize when the subject they are addressing does not lie in the domain of psychiatric competence.

Having attracted, selected, and trained students, we must admit them to the profession and monitor their performance in it. This raises issues of standards, certification, licensure, and related subjects. These have been matters of considerable public attention in recent years, but this attention has usually been addressed to protecting the public from unethical or dangerously incompetent practice, rather than improving the average or standard practice or raising the quality of the very best practice. The profession has a responsibility to pursue all of these goals. It is not always recognized that specific methods are appropriate for each of them.

Codes of professional ethics, committees reviewing allegations of malpractice or unethical conduct, and similar procedures are designed to protect the public from extraordinarily bad professional conduct. They are, for the most part, expensive and ineffective; they consume a great deal of time; most offenses are never discovered, and even when they are, the public is often poorly protected. However, they do serve one important goal: they assure the public that the profession is truly interested in public welfare rather than merely in protecting its members, and this is sufficient reason to develop and maintain them, especially since public trust is essential for professional functioning, and the public currently regards professions with considerable skepticism.

The most effective method of raising the average or standard level of professional practice is through education rather than policing, both preparatory education of students and continuing education of members of the profession. Evaluation and certification should be integrated with these educational efforts, as with all others, but without losing sight of the primary goal of the educational process: to influence attitudes, develop skills, and alter behavior. We have learned with difficulty in primary, secondary, undergraduate, and medical education that excessive attention to evaluation rather than to students and curriculum may lead to the development of students who learn to pass examinations rather than master the subject matter. It would be unfortunate if we were not able to transfer this knowledge to specialty and continuing education without repeating that experience. Methods of peer review and monitoring that contribute to the growth and education of the individual practitioner are likely to raise the general standard of professional practice; those that are experienced as disciplinary will lead to the development of skills in avoiding detection and punishment. The early efforts in this area are not totally reassuring.

Raising the level of the best professional activity requires advances in the scientific base of the profession and the translation of these advances into patterns of practice. Psychiatry has paid more attention to the speedy and effective dissemination of new knowledge than most other professions, but along with the rest of medicine it has rather passively accepted the role of commercial enterprises, with other than professional priorities, in educating psychiatrists about advances in psychiatric treatment. As our scientific knowledge grows more rapidly, the problem of disseminating new knowledge to practitioners who may not have a firm basic science foundation will become even more severe.

The final and most difficult step, after attracting, selecting, training, and monitoring members of the profession is the most painful one—removing those who are not appropriate. The profession's willingness to face this issue is a crucial factor in public trust, and to date it has not done very well. We have the right to ask respect for our titles and credentials only to the extent that we can assure that others with those titles and credentials merit equal respect. Indeed this was the origin of the earliest codes of medical ethics; peripatetic physicians policed the behavior of their colleagues so that any member of the fraternity would be recognized as worthy of trust and respect when entering a strange community. If the profession does not accept its responsibility to remove incompetent members, it will become little more than a trade union, defending the parochial interests of its members against the claims of their employers, in this case the public, while the latter will inevitably organize in an adversarial relation to the profession. This process has already begun, and it will accelerate rapidly unless the public comes to believe that it will be better protected by the profession's internal review procedures.

In addition to developing the knowledge base of the profession, and assuring the quality and quantity of its members, the profession has a responsibility to participate in distributing the scarce resources required for its work. Usually the scarcest resource is people, the members of the profession, although ancillary workers and physical facilities may be involved as well. The distribution of these resources involves their availability to all segments of the community, in terms of geography, social or economic status, age, cultural group, or degree of need. In almost every one of these respects, psychiatry has a rather poor record, although it has been improving rapidly in recent years. The profession cannot solve these problems by itself, since they often reflect general problems of resource distribution in the society or anti-professional values of certain groups. However, it has a responsibility to address itself to them and to be certain that its own contributions, whether they be patterns of training, preferred areas of inquiry, or criteria for peer recognition and approval, contribute to solutions rather than to problems.

A related type of resource distribution involves the distribution of personnel among various professional goals, such as different types of clinical care, teaching, and research. Here also the profession is only one participant in what is often a political decision-making process, but it is a critical participant. The distribution of resources among these goals involves technical questions of cost and the probability of benefit that only the profession can answer, and it involves ethical questions of balancing the interests of contemporary patients against those of future individuals who might be at risk. Psychiatrists are not more ethical than other citizens, but they should have greater understanding of their patients and more experience with the problems of the mentally ill. This circumstance often provides them with an awareness and sensitivity to related ethical questions that is not available to other citizens. To complicate the picture further, questions of resource distribution often involve balancing the career interests of one group of professionals against those of another. The optimal resolution of these complex problems cannot be assured by participation of the profession, but it is impossible without such participation.

A theme that has appeared repeatedly in this discussion is the responsibility of the profession of psychiatry to be an advisor and at times an advocate. It advises the public on scientific matters that fall within its domain, and educates the public about the extent of that domain. The latter is particularly important, since psychiatrists are experts in understanding the reasons that the public overestimates the expertise of psychiatrists. Psychiatry advises its patients. Indeed, that is its core role, and it also advocates these patients' interests in the public arena, recognizing that they may be relatively inept at doing so themselves and that the public may have more difficulty empathizing with the problems of the mentally ill than with most other disadvantaged groups. Finally, psychiatry advocates the interests of psychiatrists. This should not be concealed, but recognized as a professional responsibility rather than an embarrassing indulgence. Only a few years ago, it would have seemed silly to speak of the social value of assuring that psychiatry remain an attractive profession; today, it seems conceivable that whether or not the medical students of the future are attracted to psychiatry might become a limiting factor in the well-being of the mentally ill.

MEETING THESE RESPONSIBILITIES

How should the responsibilities of the profession be discharged? We have already spoken of the responsibility of individual psychiatrists to participate in professional activities. A corollary is that professional organizations and societies must invite this participation and provide for broad representation and democratic participation in professional decisions. A topic of growing interest is the appropriate role of nonprofessional public representation in professional decision-making. This has already begun in ethics review boards, licensure groups, and selection committees, and will probably extend further. It tends to make professional decision-making more public, and to help to differentiate the profession's self-interest from its assessment of the public interest. I believe that the profession's attitude toward this trend should be professional; that is, we should first evaluate its impact on the ability of the members of the profession to serve the public, and only secondarily consider our personal preferences or prejudices.

CONCLUSION

In summary, psychiatrists have a responsibility to participate in their profession, and psychiatry has a responsibility that extends beyond the aggregate responsibilities of individual practitioners. It must assist the public in developing new knowledge, select, train, and monitor the performance of individual psychiatrists, distribute scarce resources, advocate the interests of its patients, and conduct all of these activities in a manner that assures the public that the profession of psychiatry is interested in the public's welfare.

REFERENCES

1. Chodoff, P.: The psychiatrist's responsibility to his society. In: C. K. Hofling (Ed.), *Law and Ethics in the Practice of Psychiatry*. New York: Brunner/Mazel, 1981.
2. Freidson, E.: *Profession of Medicine.* New York: Dodd, Mead, 1973.
3. Goode, W. J.: Encroachment, charlatanism, and the emerging profession:

Psychology, medicine, and sociology. *American Sociological Review*, 25: 908-914, 1960.

4. Veatch, R. M.: Generalization of expertise. *Hastings Center Studies*, 1:29-40, 1973.

5. Hughes, E. C.: The study of occupations. In: R. Merton (Ed.), *Sociology Today*. New York: Basic Books, 1959.

6. Michels, R.: Professional ethics and social values. *The International Review of Psycho-Analysis*, 3:377-384, 1976.

7. In the service of the state: The psychiatrist as double agent. A Conference on Conflicting Loyalties. *The Hastings Center Report*, Special Supplement, 8:1-23, April, 1978.

8. Michels, R.: Ethical issues of psychological and psychotherapeutic means of behavior control. *The Hastings Center Report*, 3:11-13, 1973.

Index

warnings in, legal requirements for, 140
Nixon, Richard, 84
No-fault divorce law, 167-68
Nuclear family, 167

Obsessive-compulsive personality, 194, 217
O'Connor v. Donaldson, 12
Okpaku, Sheila, 174, 186n.
"Ordinary good parent" concept, 174
Organic brain syndrome, 159
Outpatient care and drugs, 50
Overadvocacy by expert witnesses, 163-64
Overstimulation, 195
"Overview: Ethical Issues in Contemporary Psychiatry" (Redlich and Mollica), 52

Painter v. Bannister, 172
Panic of patients, 17
Paranoia, 127
Parens patriae doctrine, 32, 36, 41
Parental-rights doctrine, xiv, 169
Parham v. J. L., 18
Parsons, T., 98, 117n.
Paternity suit, 154
Patient as Person, The (Ramsey), 52
Patient rights, 8-20, 78
  and competence, 103
  conclusion on, 19-20
  constitutional, 10, 14, 16
  movement for, 8
  and patient status, 37-38, 48-49, 60-62
  to refuse treatment, 13-19, 62
  and responsibilities, 62
  self-determination, 94, 95, 96
Peptic ulcer, 200, 201
Phrenology, 29
Physicians. *See also* Psychiatrists
  in Michigan, 183
  public obligation of, 242
Plato, 54
Poddar, Prosenjit, 119, 124, 125, 126
Poorhouses and mental hospitals, 34
Positivism, logical, and mental illness, 40

Pragmatism and mental illness, 40-41
Principles of Medical Ethics (AMA), 98, 133
Pritchard, H. A., 39
Privacy. *See* Confidentiality and privacy
Privacy Act of 1974, 78
Privacy Protection Study Commission, 78, 84
Professionalization, 239-42
Promiscuity, sexual, and children, 216
Psychiatrists:
  and behavioral scientists, 42-43
  and disclosure/consent, 100-13
  as expert witnesses, 54, 151-66
  and informal consent, 103-13
  in Michigan, 183
  need for, 244
  professional responsibilities of, 36-37, 47-48, 59-60
  professional rights of, 36, 46-47, 59
  professional split among, 236-37
  professional stance of, 35-37, 45-48, 58-59
  recruitment of, 244-45
  resource distribution of, 248-49
  scientific status of, 41
  social responsibilities of, 225-50
    citizenship, 225-28
    conclusion on, 250
    and ethics, 239-43
    public accountability, 225, 228-37
    socio-economic equity, 225, 237
  standards of, 247-48
  training of, 245-46
Psychoanalysis, 56, 101
  influence of, 43
  scientific status of, 41
  therapeutic method of, 48-49
Psychobiography, 226-27
Psychological best interests test in child custody cases, 170-71
Psychological parent, defined, 171
Psychological testimony. *See* Child custody cases
Psychopharmacology. *See* Drugs
Psychosexual development:
  and family problems, 195
  needs for normal, 196